Turmeric for Health

100 Amazing and Unexpected Uses for Turmeric

Britt Brandon, CFNS, CPT

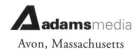
Adamsmedia
Avon, Massachusetts

Published by
Adams Media, a division of F+W Media, Inc.
57 Littlefield Street, Avon, MA 02322. U.S.A.
www.adamsmedia.com

Contains material adapted from *The Everything® Eating Clean Cookbook for Vegetarians* by Britt Brandon, copyright © 2013 by F+W Media, Inc., ISBN 10: 1-4405-5140-5, ISBN 13: 978-1-4405-5140-6; *The Everything® Healthy Green Drinks Book* by Britt Brandon, copyright © 2014 by F+W Media, Inc., ISBN 10: 1-4405-7694-7, ISBN 13: 978-1-4405-7694-2; and *The Everything® Mediterranean Cookbook, 2nd Edition* by Peter Minaki, copyright © 2013 by F+W Media, Inc., ISBN 10: 1-4405-6855-3, ISBN 13: 978-1-4405-6855-8.

ISBN 10: 1-4405-9467-8
ISBN 13: 978-1-4405-9467-0
eISBN 10: 1-4405-9468-6
eISBN 13: 978-1-4405-9468-7

Printed in the United States of America.

10 9 8 7 6 5 4 3 2 1

Library of Congress Cataloging-in-Publication Data
Brandon, Britt, author.
Turmeric for health / Britt Brandon, CFNS, CPT.
Avon, Massachusetts: Adams Media, 2016.
Includes index and bibliographical references.
LCCN 2016021760 (print) | LCCN 2016023496 (ebook) | ISBN 9781440594670 (pb) | ISBN 1440594678 (pb) | ISBN 9781440594687 (ebook) | ISBN 1440594686 (ebook)
LCSH: Turmeric--Therapeutic use. | Turmeric--Health aspects. | BISAC: HEALTH & FITNESS / Alternative Therapies. | HEALTH & FITNESS / Healing. | HEALTH & FITNESS / Beauty & Grooming.
LCC RS165.T8 B73 2016 (print) | LCC RS165.T8 (ebook) | DDC 615.3/2439--dc23
LC record available at *https://lccn.loc.gov/2016021760*

The various uses of turmeric as a health aid are based on tradition, scientific theories, or limited research. They often have not been thoroughly tested in humans, and safety and effectiveness have not yet been proven in clinical trials. Some of the conditions for which turmeric can be used as a treatment or remedy are potentially serious, and should be evaluated by a qualified healthcare provider.

This book is intended as general information only, and should not be used to diagnose or treat any health condition. In light of the complex, individual, and specific nature of health problems, this book is not intended to replace professional medical advice. The ideas, procedures, and suggestions in this book are intended to supplement, not replace, the advice of a trained medical professional. Consult your physician before adopting any of the suggestions in this book, as well as about any condition that may require diagnosis or medical attention. The author and publisher disclaim any liability arising directly or indirectly from the use of this book.

Always follow safety and commonsense cooking protocol while using kitchen utensils, operating ovens and stoves, and handling uncooked food. If children are assisting in the preparation of any recipe, they should always be supervised by an adult.

Many of the designations used by manufacturers and sellers to distinguish their products are claimed as trademarks. Where those designations appear in this book and F+W Media, Inc. was aware of a trademark claim, the designations have been printed with initial capital letters.

Cover design by Michelle Roy Kelly.
Cover image © iStockphoto.com/Melpomenem.

This book is available at quantity discounts for bulk purchases. For information, please call 1-800-289-0963.

CONTENTS

PART 2: BEAUTY 85

INTRODUCTION

Are you suffering from a lack of energy? Chronic digestive issues? Dry skin or wrinkles? Tired of buying countless over-the-counter medications and creams that don't even seem to work? It turns out that the solution to these problems and more has been around for thousands of years: turmeric!

Turmeric is a perennial root, closely related to the well-known gingerroot, that has traveled from the coasts of South Asia across the globe to grace the entire world with delicious flavors and immense health benefits. With its distinctive peppery, warm, earthy flavoring, it has improved the taste and aroma of dishes that are now craved across continents. While turmeric has been used for medicinal properties in the Asian countries for thousands of years, only recently have the Americas embraced the natural healing capabilities of turmeric. It's not just for making mustard! Because it contains vitamins, minerals, and unique phytochemicals that make this specific spice an effective alternative to pharmaceutical and over-the-counter remedies, turmeric is able to improve and transform health and well-being—naturally.

Turmeric has been shown to be an effective reliever of nausea, diarrhea, and inadequate nutrient absorption, and can even combat symptoms associated with chemotherapy. While preventing illnesses and promoting health throughout the body, turmeric also enhances brain health, helping to improve memory, fight Alzheimer's disease, and reduce or eliminate symptoms associated with Parkinson's and multiple sclerosis, all while protecting the brain and nervous system from potentially cancerous changes within brain cells that can lead to catastrophic (and possibly fatal!) developments.

The health benefits don't stop with the positive influences on overall health aspects, either—skin, hair, and nails also benefit from simple-to-create mixtures that incorporate turmeric. In this book, you'll find step-by-step instructions for such mixtures, plus numerous recipes for delicious dishes that include turmeric so your taste buds can benefit from the savory spice as well.

The National Center for Complementary and Integrative Health estimates that Americans spend more than $30 billion in the complementary and alternative medicine industry every year. With the overwhelming number of products and options out there, you need to know which products really work so you can spend your money wisely! Let turmeric, an affordable and easy-to-use choice, lead the way. Every page of this book will show you how to create and combine beneficial remedies and applications that will transform your life naturally . . . inside and out!

TURMERIC'S MANY HEALTH BENEFITS

What Is Turmeric?

Used internationally as a staple spice in cuisine, an element of holistic medicine, an offering in religious ceremonies, and even a coloring in cosmetics, turmeric has been providing the world with countless uses and immense health benefits for thousands of years. The scientific name for the plant is *Curcuma longa*, a well-known perennial belonging to the ginger family of Zingiberaceae. The adult plant produces the turmeric offshoot roots that can grow up to 1 meter in height. With beautiful long, oblong leaves, this precious plant is known to have more than 133 species worldwide.

Turmeric's beautiful bright yellow root has led to its nicknames "the golden spice" and "Indian saffron." It has graced countless cultures around the world with its gorgeous coloring, unique aroma, and unmistakable flavor. Available in a natural state of the whole root or in powdered, pressed, or extract forms, turmeric can provide countless preventative and healing measures.

A Brief History

Native to the southwest of India, turmeric has been a staple of Ayurvedic medicine for more than 4,000 years. Its use has spread recently around the world to contribute to the healing and preventative medicinal applications of countless conditions. Around c.e. 700, the turmeric plant is thought to have arrived in China. The earliest record of the plant is in one of the first Ayurvedic scientific and medical documents, the Sanskrit text *Compendium of Caraka* (written between the fourth century b.c.e. and the second century c.e.), which recommended turmeric as an efficient remedy for food poisoning. Marco Polo later recorded references to the beauty and importance of turmeric in 1280 as he traveled around the world.

Turmeric became a staple of the culture and cuisine of India, where they utilized the root for multiple applications. People in India became such devout believers in the root's healing and protective powers that they became planters and suppliers; India now produces more than 80 percent of the world's turmeric. The Indian city of Erode, commonly referred to as "The Yellow City," is known for growing turmeric with the highest concentration of its profound phytochemical, curcumin.

While cultures worldwide have been using turmeric for centuries, countries geared more toward administering "modern" pharmaceutical medicines have only been studying turmeric's effectiveness in recent years. With more than 3,000 studies published in peer-reviewed journals in the last twenty-five years showing the amazing benefits of turmeric, turmeric has made quite an entrance into the Western medicinal world.

Turmeric's Unique Chemical Profile

Turmeric contains more than 100 astounding chemical compounds that contribute to its ability to help treat conditions from stomachaches to respiratory illness. These chemical compounds are what make turmeric unique. Most importantly, turmeric contains curcumin, which is a polyphenol. Polyphenols are organic chemicals that have been shown to have anti-inflammatory properties. Polyphenols are also present in other foods and beverages, such as epigallocatechin in green tee, capsaicin in chili peppers, and resveratrol in red wine and fresh peanuts. Curcumin is what gives turmeric its beautiful yellow-orange color. Curcuminoids, the group of chemical compounds in turmeric, include curcumin, demethoxycurcumin, and bisdemethoxycurcumin. Turmeric also contains volatile oils, including tumerone, artumerone, and zingiberene. Curcumin is the part of turmeric that has been studied most frequently for its uses as a dietary supplement and in food coloring and cosmetics. One study conducted by the Asian Coordinating Group for Chemistry showed that turmeric extracts may have antifungal and antibacterial properties. The National Institutes of Health lists more than eighty studies that are looking into turmeric's ability to treat and heal issues, from irritable bowel syndrome to diabetic nephropathy. (Visit *https://clinicaltrials.gov* for updated information on these studies.)

Turmeric's unique chemical composition of vitamins, minerals, fiber, and phytochemicals provide the body with:

- Promotion of immunity
- Protection against illness and disease
- Prevention of the development of serious illness and disease
- Destruction of chronic disease cells within the brain and body

Thanks to these properties, turmeric has now been integrated into natural treatment methods for common and chronic conditions.

The Special Benefits of Turmeric

The turmeric root possesses natural oils, amino acids, vitamins, minerals, fatty acids, and phytochemicals that combine to provide healing properties for almost every area of the body. Phytochemicals are naturally occurring plant compounds that boost the healthy functioning of cells, tissues, organs, and systems. These compounds include antioxidants, anti-inflammatory agents, analgesics, and a wide variety of protective, preventative, and health-promoting derivatives that help support the natural functions of the body. The powerful phenols contained within the flesh of the turmeric root are varieties of curcuminoids: curcumin, desmethoxycurcumin, and bisdesmethoxycurcumin, which not only help combat germs, bacteria, and viruses but also help aid in digestive processes, support immunity, improve energy, maximize metabolic functioning, cleanse the blood, regulate blood sugar, and increase mental processes.

We'll go into more depth on the benefits of turmeric throughout this book, but here is some basic information on turmeric's powerful nutrients.

Vitamins

The vitamins obtained through food help support every organ, system, and function in the body. With each vitamin delivering energy, improving immunity, protecting cell health, and maintaining proper metabolic functioning, it's easy to see why these nutrients are essential and why avoiding a deficiency of any vitamin is crucial to maintaining overall health. Turmeric provides a number of essential vitamins and also contains natural oils and enzymes that improve the body's ability to absorb, process, and utilize vitamins for maximum benefits. The vitamins provided by turmeric include:

- *Vitamin A*: essential for vision health and prevention of cataracts. Vitamin A also helps with the formation of hormones; contributes to the maintenance of teeth, tissue, and cell membrane health; works to maintain healthy hair production; and prevents oxidative activity in cells that can destroy cell health or transform cells to cancerous copies of themselves.
- *B Vitamins*: essential energy-boosting vitamins that contribute to muscle health and assist in protein synthesis and the metabolism of all nutrients throughout the body. Certain B vitamins can also prevent neural-tube defects in fetuses and promote healthy brain functioning, and are required for the formation of blood cells and DNA.
- *Vitamin C*: antiviral agent and powerful antioxidant that prevents oxidative and free-radical activity in cells, which can turn healthy cells to damaged cells responsible for the development of serious illnesses and diseases like cancer. Vitamin C is required for the absorption and use of iron, calcium, and folate; helps build and maintain healthy bones, teeth, gums, and blood vessels; assists in wound and bruise healing; and fights infection. This vitamin cannot be stored in the body and must therefore be regularly consumed in appropriate amounts.
- *Vitamin E*: powerful antioxidant that acts to promote the health of cells by protecting against oxidative damage caused by free radicals. Also helping to support neurological functioning throughout the body, vitamin E is essential for enzymatic reactions and communication between the nervous system and the brain.
- *Vitamin K*: needed in adequate stores for calcification of the bones; inadequate amounts of this nutrient can result in brittle bones and even unhealthy teeth. Vitamin K is also an essential part of the protein synthesis process that is required for proper blood processes such as coagulation, which helps to reduce the risk of excessive bleeding.

Minerals

Minerals are essential nutrients, obtained from foods, that help support the structures and processes in the body. Contributing to the health of the bones, teeth, hair, skin, and nails, minerals also maintain the health of the heart, brain, and digestive system by cleansing the blood, improving nerve health, boosting immunity, and upholding the heart and cardiovascular system's strength. The minerals provided by turmeric include:

- *Calcium*: aids in the cell's absorption of nutrients; is required for muscle contractions that allow us to move, jump, exercise, and also pump blood throughout the heart and body; promotes proper blood clotting; supports bone health; is essential for proper nerve functioning and communication; is required for insulin production and secretion; improves immune system functioning by playing a role in the enzymatic reactions of T cells in the immune system; is involved in the production of white blood cells; and promotes healthy sleep.
- *Iron*: improves immune system functioning; promotes brain functioning, mental clarity, and energy; fights fatigue; increases the body's absorption of vitamin C.
- *Magnesium*: supports bone health; is required for the formation of cells; is involved in protein absorption, production, and use; assists in the body's absorption and use of B vitamins; promotes energy production and insulin production and secretion; improves nervous system functioning; is involved in muscle repair; and assists in the absorption of calcium, vitamin C, and potassium.
- *Manganese*: is required for the enzymatic reactions that take place in the body for hormone production, energy use, and a number of metabolic processes; regulates blood sugar levels; improves metabolic functioning; and is essential for the production of thyroid hormones.
- *Phosphorous*: combines with calcium to promote the healthy formation of bones and teeth, and promotes healthy nervous system functioning.
- *Potassium*: promotes proper growth of the body's bones, muscles, and tissues; maintains healthy fluid balance within cells; prevents muscle cramping; promotes healthy kidney functioning and cardiovascular system functioning (specifically required for the maintenance of a healthy heartbeat); and

supports the respiratory system by strengthening the lungs and improving the processes related to breathing and processing oxygen.

- *Sodium*: regulates blood pressure, regulates fluid balance within cells and throughout the body, and is required for the healthy functioning of the nerves and muscles.
- *Zinc*: required for the metabolism of proteins and carbohydrates, promotes healthy immune system functioning, and supports wound healing and eye health.

Turmeric also contains quercetin, a plant pigment that gives many fruits and vegetables their color. They are antioxidants, scavenging free radicals, which can damage cells.

When to Be Careful with Turmeric

Turmeric is generally a very safe ingredient and supplement. However, talk with your doctor before beginning any routine that includes it. Here are some specific situations that require extra attention before using turmeric:

- Eating turmeric in foods is safe during pregnancy, but turmeric supplements may not be.
- Those with gallbladder problems might find that turmeric exacerbates them.
- Turmeric might slow blood clotting, so those with bleeding problems or an upcoming surgery should be cautious.
- Curcumin might decrease blood sugar in diabetics.
- High amounts of turmeric might affect iron absorption.
- Turmeric might decrease testosterone levels and sperm movement, which could affect fertility.
- High levels of turmeric might increase the production of stomach acid, which could be problematic for those with reflux or ulcers.

How to Select, Store, and Prepare

There are many options for integrating turmeric into your health and beauty regimens. You'll find over-the-counter supplements at local drugstores or natural health food stores. The best supplements will contain 95 percent curcuminoids and be void of preservatives, artificial ingredients, and dyes. For the best supplements, search online for an up-to-date list of independently tested supplements that meet or exceed industry standards.

Fresh turmeric can be kept on your countertop or in the fridge or freezer, ready to be freshly prepared any time, any day, for up to two weeks! You'll usually buy the root, which is yellow and resembles a gingerroot but is bright orange-yellow under the skin. It has a warm, peppery flavor and mild fragrance. As with any fresh root, you can shred, chop, cook, or dry it, giving yourself lots of ways to incorporate the flavors and nutritional benefits into your daily routine. You can include turmeric simply and easily in your everyday life using these delicious variations:

- *Chopped*: Ideal for purées, smoothies, simple cooked dishes, or roasting. The root itself is very dense but is easily steamed when combined with meats, vegetables, or oils. Simply peel the exterior of the root, cut off both ends, and slice the root lengthwise into two symmetrical pieces. Now chop into pieces of desired thickness. You can roast a pan of these chopped pieces, tossed in olive oil to coat, at a temperature of 350°F for 30 minutes, turning every 10–15 minutes until soft.
- *Sliced*: Ideal for purées, smoothies, and simple dishes. Extremely thin slices can even be used as a beautiful garnish. Beware that roasting may take more time for thicker cut pieces. Peel the exterior of the root, cut off both ends, and slice the root to produce slices of desired thickness.
- *Powdered*: Powdered turmeric is not difficult to make and is very useful for smoothies, slow-cooker recipes, and stir-fries. Regularly available at grocery stores, powdered turmeric can be purchased and stored for everyday use in a cool, dark pantry. If you prefer to make your own powdered turmeric at home, the process (while a bit lengthy, becomes easier with practice) involves peeling the exterior of the root, chopping it into similarly sized ¼" pieces, and placing the pieces into a pot large enough to cover them with 4" of water. Cover the pot with a tight-fitting lid, and bring to a rolling boil over high heat. Reduce heat to low, and continue to simmer until roots are

tender. Remove from heat, drain, place roots on dry towels, and allow to set in the sun for 10–12 days until shrunken and browned. Use a food processor to blend the dried roots to a fine powder. Move to an airtight container, and store in a low-humidity area that is dark and free from natural light. Homemade powdered turmeric will keep for about 3–6 months in these conditions.

- *Pressed/Supplement*: Pressed forms of powdered turmeric are readily available and can easily be taken to consume the recommended dosage for the ideal health goal you wish to reach. By visiting major online distributors (such as Amazon.com or one of the numerous distributors of organically grown turmeric who help educated consumers purchase high-quality products) and by monitoring the manufacturer's history, reputation, and approval rating, you can easily research companies to ensure your organic turmeric is authentic.
- *Aerosol*: Turmeric's main powerhouse, curcumin, is also available as an aerosol that you can spray directly into your mouth to inhale. This method might help make curcumin even more bioavailable to the body than ingestion.
- *Extract/Tincture*: You can find turmeric tinctures at health food stores, vitamin outlets, and online. They usually have an herb to alcohol ratio of 1:2. The tincture form of turmeric extract can deliver turmeric's anti-inflammatory polyphenols (such as 1-alpha-curcumene, 1-beta-curcumene, camphene, and camphor) directly to the bloodstream through the skin. With antioxidant benefits that provide protection against illness and disease, prevent dangerous cellular changes, and promote the functioning of the body's organs and systems, turmeric tincture is readily used among cultures all over the world.

Incorporating turmeric into your daily routines couldn't be easier. Let's delve into 100 ways this natural root and spice can treat common conditions that have plagued people worldwide for centuries.

PART 1

HEALTH

If you're on a quest to achieve optimal health, you're probably over-whelmed by all the options available. Turmeric allows you to stay simple and natural in your efforts to meet your health and fitness goals. Scientific studies have recently shed light on the importance of attaining protective nutrients from whole foods, so spices like turmeric are a perfect option. Whether you find yourself plagued with sleepless nights, nutrient deficiency, chronic illnesses, or serious disease, the implementation of turmeric can help improve your health.

With essential B vitamins; vitamins A, C, D, and E; and miner-als like iron, potassium, magnesium, and manganese (just to name a few!), turmeric can contribute important nutrients of all kinds to your daily diet. Because it also contains potent phytochemicals that are unique to this worldly spice, turmeric works to improve the nutrition content of your daily diet routine so you can maxi-mize benefits to your health . . . all with a simple 2-tablespoon serving per day.

The teas, tinctures, and dishes in this section will add flavor-ful depth to any recipe, reduce tummy troubles, and regulate your blood sugar! It's time to start seeing your health improve—natu-rally and deliciously.

1. ADDS MANGANESE TO THE DIET

Manganese, a trace mineral usually obtained through plant-based dietary sources, helps to improve bone quality and strength. Manganese also helps activate enzymes like prolidase—which helps make collagen, a structural component of skin—and helps protect skin from UV rays.

The body does not naturally store much manganese, so it's good to take a supplement to maximize manganese's health benefits. It's also helpful to add manganese-rich foods, like turmeric, cloves, dark leafy greens, oats, and root vegetables, to your diet.

A 2-teaspoon serving of powdered turmeric contains 17 percent of the daily recommended intake of manganese. Add at least 2 teaspoons of grated, powdered, or fresh turmeric to your meals, snacks, and drinks daily to ensure your body can reap all of the amazing benefits that manganese provides.

TO MAKE A MANGANESE-RICH SMOOTHIE, COMBINE:

1 cup chopped spinach

1 medium yam, cut into pieces

1 medium red apple, cored

2 teaspoons turmeric

2. BOOSTS IRON INTAKE

If you've ever experienced unusual fatigue, weakness, pale skin, brittle nails, and dizziness, an iron deficiency could have been the cause. Iron is found within the ground, as well as in green leafy vegetables, fermented curds like tofu, and meats, and is the number one essential mineral required by the body. Almost three-quarters of the iron in your body is found in the red blood cells (hemoglobin) and muscle cells (myoglobin). Iron is required for a number of important biochemical reactions that take place every second of every day, such as:

■ Transferring oxygen in the blood to lungs and tissues
■ Producing thyroid hormones
■ Supporting the health of neurotransmitters, which facilitate communication among nerve cells
■ Strengthening the immune system

If you find yourself falling a bit short in the daily recommendation of iron, you could take an iron supplement—but many people report unpleasant side effects of constipation and cramping. Instead, try turmeric! Turmeric boasts a high content of naturally derived iron—approximately 15 percent of the daily recommended intake in 1 tablespoon! To up your iron intake, add turmeric to your favorite dishes, smoothies, or salads, or take it as a simple supplement.

3. PROVIDES KEY B VITAMINS

B vitamins are known as the "happy vitamins" because of their countless health benefits and because a vitamin-B deficiency can contribute to emotional disturbances. Mood fluctuations, irritability, dips in energy, and mental "fogginess" can be attributed to inadequate vitamin B intake.

There are eight B vitamins:

- B_1 (Thiamine)
- B_2 (Riboflavin)
- B_3 (Niacin)
- B_5 (Pantothenic Acid)
- B_6 (Pyridoxine)
- B_7 (Biotin)
- B_9 (Folic Acid)
- B_{12} (Cobalamin)

All of the B vitamins work hand in hand with one another and with the other essential vitamins and minerals in the diet to ensure that the body and brain function properly. Known for aiding the brain's production of the biochemicals serotonin and dopamine, B vitamins may help maintain a balanced mood. These Bs are also able to:

- Improve healthy brain functioning (like memory and focus)
- Ensure proper production and maintenance of red blood cells
- Aid reproductive processes
- Support healthy growth and development, even in infants and small children

One B vitamin in particular (folic acid) is commonly prescribed to pregnant women in early pregnancy for its ability to help avoid a condition known as *spina bifida*, in which a child is born without a completely developed spinal covering.

Turmeric can be an excellent supplement for people who adhere to a meat-free diet since meats and meat products can contain a great amount of B vitamins. Ground turmeric contains a good amount of B_6 in particular—a 2-teaspoon serving contains approximately 5 percent of the daily recommended intake.

4. INCREASES POTASSIUM INTAKE

Potassium is a unique mineral because it does double-duty as both a mineral and an electrolyte. This powerful essential helps the body in both cellular and electrical productions and processes, and is known for being one of the most soluble minerals (meaning it can easily be dissolved and absorbed by the body with minimal effort). The body relies on potassium, the primary positive ion in cells, to ensure proper development, functioning, and processing of biochemical reactions and protein synthesis.

Potassium also contributes to the supporting processes involved in proper metabolic functioning and energy production by being an essential part of the process of breaking down carbohydrates, converting them to glucose and storing them as glycogen for future energy use.

The symptoms of deficiencies in potassium can vary widely from person to person, but they most commonly include negative effects on the heart, blood flow, and communication between neurotransmitters in the brain and throughout the body. Symptoms like fatigue, lack of focus, poor memory, high blood pressure/hypertension, failure to thrive or grow properly, slow reaction time, and muscle weakness are all examples of potassium-deficiency symptoms. A 2-teaspoon serving of ground turmeric provides approximately 3 percent of the daily recommended intake of potassium.

5. SUPPLY MUCH-NEEDED FIBER

The most widely accepted recommendation for daily fiber intake looms around the 25–30 gram per day range, yet most people don't get anywhere near that amount. That's why you see fiber supplements in countless forms in drugstore aisles across the country. Over-the-counter fiber supplements are available in powders, pills, and drinks, but can also bombard your body with synthetic additives that are either unnecessary or unhealthy. If you want to improve your daily fiber intake naturally, shift your diet to whole, natural foods like fruits, vegetables, and whole grains. You can easily acquire the necessary amounts of fiber if your diet is filled with these foods. Fiber helps your body in countless ways, such as:

■ Fighting cravings naturally because fiber provides more satiety at meals
■ Improving digestive processing and nutrient absorption
■ Keeping stools soft and preventing constipation
■ Promoting healthy bacterial growth and cleansing within the colon (helping to fend off serious complications and even cancers)
■ Maintaining higher energy levels throughout the day because fiber

balances blood sugars for extended periods (bye-bye, midday slump!)

If you find yourself searching for great dietary additions that can add daily doses of fiber to your diet naturally, turmeric is a delicious spice and ingredient that can help ensure you're consuming enough fiber throughout the day. A 2-teaspoon serving provides about 4 percent of the daily recommended intake of fiber.

TO MAKE A MEAL WITH FIBER AND TURMERIC, FOLLOW THESE INSTRUCTIONS:

2 tablespoons extra-virgin olive oil
1 cup carrot matchsticks
1 cup chopped celery
½ cup chopped onion
½ cup thinly sliced red pepper
1 tablespoon powdered turmeric
1 teaspoon salt
½ teaspoon garlic powder
2 chicken breasts, halved and cut into ¼" strips
½ zucchini, halved and sliced thin
¼ cup vegetable broth
¼ cup Greek yogurt
2 cups cooked rice

In a large sauté pan over medium heat, drizzle oil and swirl to coat pan evenly. Add carrots, celery, onions, and red peppers, and sprinkle with turmeric, salt, and garlic powder. Cook for 3–4 minutes until vegetables are slightly softened.

Add chicken and zucchini and cook for 5–7 minutes, turning consistently until chicken is cooked through.

Add vegetable broth to pan gradually, mixing chicken and vegetables to coat. Remove from heat.

Cool for 5 minutes before adding yogurt, mixing in to coat chicken and vegetables evenly. Serve ¼ of chicken and vegetable curry mixture over ¼ cup rice. (Serves 4.)

RECOMMENDATIONS FOR USE:

Utilize naturally fiber-rich turmeric in a variety of dishes and snacks to boost flavor *and* add natural benefits to your health as well.

6. REGULATES BLOOD SUGAR

When so many body processes, functions, and procedures are dependent upon consistent levels of blood sugar, it's no wonder the topic has become a major concern in the health world. A growing number of patients are dealing with blood sugar issues every day. From a lack of focus or dips in energy levels to constant fatigue or complications from obesity, the symptoms of erratic blood sugar levels can be nothing short of life altering. More and more people with type 2 diabetes turn to synthetic forms of insulin, a hormone that should be naturally produced by the body to correct its sugar imbalance. With a focus on natural foods that are fiber-rich with stable supplies of carbohydrates, sugars, and fats that can all work synergistically to regulate blood sugar, anyone can transform their health and reduce the signs and symptoms of poor blood sugar control.

Turmeric has been studied by countless researchers around the globe to see if the spice's main chemical compound, curcuminoids, could assist in regulating blood sugar levels . . . and the results have consistently shown that it can—naturally! A related study published in *Diabetes Care*, a magazine published by the American Diabetes Association, considered 240 patients who met the American Diabetes Association's criteria for prediabetes. None of those who took curcumin developed prediabetes, while 16 percent of their placebo counterparts did. With an intake of only 300 mg per day, patients have shown success in reducing their requirement for blood-sugar-regulating medications, and have reported a reduction in symptoms that they had experienced consistently prior to the trial.

7. ADDS ZINC TO THE DIET

Coming in at a close second to iron for being the most important mineral required by the body for a myriad of processes, zinc is an essential dietary element. Zinc deficiencies can easily result in minor and serious health issues and complications, such as hair loss, poor appetite, and slowed wound healing. Zinc helps your body:

- Improve immune system functioning
- Enhance production and delivery of insulin
- Optimize cardiovascular functioning
- Complete cell division and production processes
- Break down carbohydrates
- Ensure the senses of smell and taste remain intact

Clearly, zinc is a dietary element that is an absolute must when planning your meals with a focus on achieving and maintaining optimal health.

Turmeric has been given little credit for its ability to boost your zinc intake. Adding just 2 teaspoons of powdered turmeric to your meals, snacks, or smoothies gives you 2 percent of your daily recommended intake of zinc.

TO MAKE A VEGETABLE SOUP THAT'S LOADED WITH ZINC, FOLLOW THESE INSTRUCTIONS:

1 tablespoon extra-virgin olive oil
½ cup chopped yellow onion
½ cup diced carrots
½ cup diced celery
2 cloves garlic, minced
2 teaspoons dried Italian seasoning
2 teaspoons turmeric
1 bay leaf
2 cups dry lentils
4 cups vegetable stock
4 cups water
2 large tomatoes, peeled, cored, and chopped
½ cup baby spinach leaves, rinsed
1 teaspoon all-natural sea salt
½ teaspoon cracked black pepper

Pour olive oil into a large pot over medium heat. After oil runs thin, add the onion, carrot, celery, and sauté for 5 minutes, or until tender but not burned. Add the garlic, Italian seasoning, turmeric, and bay leaf and sauté for about 1 minute before adding the lentils, stock, water, and tomatoes.

Bring pot to a boil, reduce heat, and simmer soup uncovered for about 1 hour.

Before removing from heat, add spinach, salt, and pepper. Stir until spinach is wilted. (Serves 8.)

8. STIMULATES SENSATIONS OF SATIETY

Three of turmeric's potent phytochemical compounds (curcumin, quercetin, and p-coumaric acid) provide the body with an abundance of benefits . . . one being increased sensations of satiety at mealtime. As foods are consumed throughout the day, blood sugar levels rise and fall. Insulin resistance, which can lead to type 2 diabetes, is a condition in which the body can't respond properly to the insulin it makes. Diabetes can sometimes be improved with a diet focused on low-glycemic foods that add essential vitamins and minerals to the daily diet. Lowering insulin resistance, just one of turmeric's benefits, leads to the blood sugar control that allows you to experience sustained energy and fewer energy slumps. Turmeric's healthy doses of vitamins, minerals, and fiber all support the natural processes associated with the brain and digestive system's communication, so your meals leave you feeling full and focused for a longer duration.

Overeating has become a common occurrence for the average American, leading to an emphasis on portion sizes and contents of daily meals. Instead of turning to synthetic appetite suppressants or even surgeries to avoid overeating, simply add turmeric to your meals to feel fuller faster and for longer . . . naturally!

9. ALLEVIATES HEARTBURN

Did you know that more than 60 million Americans experience heartburn at least once per month and, of that number, more than 15 million experience the condition daily? This excruciating condition, characterized as an intense burning feeling in the chest, is most commonly due to a handful of scenarios that pertain to diet, lifestyle, age, or illness. For the millions of people who have to endure heartburn on a regular basis, most are aware that evading fatty foods, abstaining from alcohol and caffeine, and refraining from smoking all help to reduce the symptoms, but for those who abide by these rules and still experience the condition, turmeric can help.

Turmeric contains anti-inflammatory compounds that have been researched in America, as well as countless countries around the globe. A study in the journal *Systematic Reviews* showed that eating 1 gram of turmeric (about 1 teaspoon) twice per day had a remarkable impact on the esophagus and colon, helping patients recover faster from indigestion. The potent compounds in turmeric also relieve the underlying issues of acid and bile overproduction, thereby promoting benefits to the body instead of painful conditions and helping to produce good bacteria, minimize bad bacteria, and improve the colon's ability to absorb beneficial nutrients.

10. REDUCES STOMACH PAIN

Stomach pain can be a debilitating condition, leaving you feeling anything from slightly queasy to doubled over in pain from extreme, intense bouts of cramping that limit movements and impair your ability to function normally. With so many possible causes of stomach pain, you should first identify whether or not the pain is resulting from a serious medical condition. If you find yourself dealing with chronic stomach pain that is constant; lasts for an extended period of time; or is accompanied by fever, dizziness, or fatigue, consult a physician immediately to rule out possible serious or life-threatening medical conditions. Irritable bowel syndrome (IBS), colitis, diverticulitis, and even cancer are just a few of the serious conditions that require medical attention and treatment.

If you are one of the millions of Americans who experience intermittent or mild stomach pain, however, the causes are more likely to be connected to diet or lifestyle. Even though mild stomach pain is less serious than the chronic alternatives, the pain can still be uncomfortable and distracting. Mild stomach pain is often caused by:

- Certain diet choices, like fattening, spicy, or even poorly prepared foods (commonly resulting in food poisoning)
- Smoking
- Alcohol consumption
- Inactivity

Luckily, turmeric contains the naturally occurring polyphenols and compounds that can aid in relieving the stomach discomfort caused by each and every one of these examples. Turmeric contains anti-inflammatory, antibacterial, antiviral, and antiparasitic compounds that can quickly alleviate your pain and get you back to feeling yourself quickly and naturally.

TO MAKE A STOMACH PAIN–REDUCING DRINK, COMBINE:

1 tablespoon grated turmeric
8 ounces hot water

RECOMMENDATIONS FOR USE:

Strain (to remove any bits of turmeric), and drink daily.

11. MINIMIZE BOUTS OF DIARRHEA

Diarrhea is an unpleasant condition, to say the least. Diarrhea's quick onset can cause the urgent need to use the restroom at any time, day or night, making it embarrassing and uncomfortable. Serious bouts of diarrhea that last for more than three days should be addressed by a medical professional to ensure the underlying cause isn't a serious condition. Most people experience occasional diarrhea, consisting of three or more loose stools in one day. It's commonly due to reactions to certain medications, intolerance of certain foods or preparation methods, food contamination, allergies, bacteria, viruses, or even stress or alcohol.

By using a combination of treatment methods along with turmeric, you can naturally calm your diarrhea and return your stools to normal while optimizing your health and protecting against diarrhea in the future. These tips can help you treat and prevent diarrhea:

- Hydrate yourself with a minimum of eight 8-ounce glasses of water per day (more when experiencing diarrhea).
- Opt for more natural, whole-food choices in your daily diet routine.
- Wash your hands frequently.
- Consume 1 teaspoon powdered turmeric up to 3 times daily when experiencing diarrhea.

Because it contains a variety of vitamins and phytochemicals that improve digestion and immunity, as well as minerals like potassium and magnesium to help with dehydration and fluid balance in the body, turmeric can improve your overall health and minimize the duration and frequency of your experiences with diarrhea . . . effectively and naturally!

12. LESSEN FLATULENCE

An uncomfortable topic of conversation, flatulence is an even more uncomfortable experience to endure. Embarrassing and unpleasant, flatulence (more commonly referred to as *gas*) can be caused by a number of factors and can strike at any time. Because gas is normally accompanied by bloating due to the entrapment of air within the digestive tract, this condition can be uncomfortable, and it can lead to minimal or extreme stomach pain and cramping. Not surprisingly, gas is normally the result of diet, so the preventative measures to avoid gas would be to avoid fatty, processed foods and dairy products (if you have a sensitivity to lactose) and focus on a diet rich in natural whole foods such as fruits, vegetables, and whole grains. Some whole foods do increase gas production, however, so if you have frequent problems with flatulence, you might want to steer clear of cruciferous vegetables, sweet fruits, and beans, as these foods can actually contribute to the development of gas.

For fast flatulence relief, turmeric can be used as an effective, all-natural remedy that's not only able to treat the symptoms of gas but the underlying issues as well . . . all while optimizing your overall health and well-being! Nourishing the entire digestive tract and improving the actual process of digestion, turmeric's polyphenols work to support enzymatic processes and alleviate the overproduction of acids that can create gas. Because it minimizes gas production, turmeric can safely, quickly, and effectively prevent and cure flatulence.

TO MAKE A GAS-REDUCING DRINK, COMBINE:

1 tablespoon grated or powdered turmeric
8 ounces water, juice, or super smoothie

RECOMMENDATIONS FOR USE:

Drink daily while experiencing gas.

13. HELPS IBS

Irritable bowel syndrome (also known as IBS) strikes millions of people each and every year. While similar and often grouped with IBS, Crohn's Disease emulates the same symptoms as IBS but leaves the patient with ongoing symptoms that are difficult to treat and control without medication. IBS, on the other hand, can be treated with changes in diet and lifestyle. For IBS sufferers, the most commonly reported symptoms are abdominal pain, irregular bowel movements, cramping, bloating, gas, and food intolerances. The condition is diagnosed if sufferers report experiencing a number of the symptoms at least three times per month for six months or more. While there is no known definitive cause of IBS, bacterial infections, viral infections, disruptive hormone levels, or even bacterial overgrowth can all contribute to the development of the condition. Your doctor might prescribe medications to treat IBS, but you might also want to supplement with a proven natural remedy: turmeric!

Packed with plentiful vitamins, minerals, and phytochemicals— including curcumin—turmeric combats digestive issues, reduces inflammation, and fights viral and bacterial infections, all while boosting immunity, improving hormonal balance, and naturally nourishing the very organs affected by IBS. Simply consume 1 tablespoon of grated, powdered, or liquid turmeric extract per day to fend off IBS symptoms while delivering natural nutrition to your entire body and brain.

14. COMBATS NAUSEA

Because a number of conditions—hunger, dehydration, illness, infection, stomach pain, anxiety, stress, and even pregnancy—are commonly associated with nausea, it can be difficult to identify the underlying cause, therefore making it difficult to treat. Many over-the-counter medications promise to treat nausea, but these medications can be packed with synthetic or unsafe ingredients like charcoal that can either fail to relieve the nausea or exacerbate the underlying issue. Natural treatments are a great option for intestinal issues like nausea because they are gentle but effective. Turmeric (and its 4,000-year history in alternative medicine as an intestinal treatment aid) comes to the rescue, with effective nutrients that not only provide nausea relief but soothe the underlying issues as well.

Curcumin is responsible for turmeric's effectiveness in the treatment of intestinal issues because of its ability to fight inflammation, microbes, bacteria, and viruses, all of which could cause feelings of nausea. But turmeric goes beyond that as well, providing vitamins, minerals, and phytochemicals that combine to act as antioxidants against illness and to promote healthy brain chemistry. Turmeric can help ease your nausea, whether it's due to a physical trigger, like food intake, *or* a mental cause, like anxiety or stress.

TO MAKE AN ANTINAUSEA DRINK, COMBINE:

1 teaspoon powdered turmeric
1 teaspoon grated ginger
8 ounces water, tea, or almond or coconut milk

RECOMMENDATIONS FOR USE:

Drink 1–3 times daily when nauseated.

15. ENCOURAGES PROPER DIGESTION

Your digestive system consists of multiple parts that work together to move and process the food you eat. From the saliva in the mouth (which starts the dissolution of food) to the muscle movements of the esophagus (which pull food into the intestines) to the release of bile by the gallbladder (which breaks down food), digestion is an intricate process. Because there are so many organs and functions involved in digestion, the process can easily be disrupted, especially if you don't get enough of the vitamins and minerals that are necessary to support those organs and their functions. The enzymes, acids, and excretions that are needed for digestion to be performed properly are only produced when adequate amounts of the nutrients they depend on are provided in the diet. Since most people find it difficult to adhere to a squeaky-clean diet of whole fruits, vegetables, lean meats, and grains to ensure maximum nutrient availability, you will be happy to discover that turmeric can help.

With turmeric's assortment of fiber, vitamins, minerals, antioxidants, and anti-inflammatory compounds, it can deliver the precise nutrition the digestive system needs to support enzymatic reactions, acid production, muscle movement, and optimal nutrient absorption. Just add 1 tablespoon of grated, powdered, or liquid turmeric extract to one of your dishes every day. All of turmeric's benefits combine to create the perfect digestive system elements that promote optimal (and regular!) digestion each and every day!

16. IMPROVES METABOLIC FUNCTIONING

Your metabolism runs on a multitude of processes that coordinate to produce the energy that the body needs to move muscles, regulate the heartbeat, support respiratory functions, and perform brain functions. These processes ensure the body efficiently processes the calories it needs to use as fuel and utilizes those calories to perform the daily functions that require that fuel. Optimal metabolic functioning leads to optimal health, with:

- High, sustained energy levels that lead to fat loss and retained muscle
- A properly performing digestive system
- Optimal hormone production
- Increased immunity

Poor metabolic functioning, on the other hand, can lead to a life of obesity, digestive issues, constant fatigue, hormonal imbalance, and even depression. So, you can easily see why ensuring top-notch metabolic functioning is so important.

Again, turmeric can help! How? Turmeric adds a flavor-packed kick to any dishes throughout your day and can help support your metabolic functioning, too. It provides vitamins, minerals, and phytochemicals that promote blood health and oxygen transport, assist with respiratory and cardiovascular functioning, and help regulate blood sugar and hormone production, all while improving energy levels and assisting in the processes involved in the breakdown and utilization of fats, proteins, and carbohydrates for proper use throughout the body. Add anywhere from 1 teaspoon to 1 tablespoon of turmeric in its grated, powdered, or extract forms to your meals to help improve your metabolic function.

17. PROMOTES FAT LOSS

The body requires specific nutrients to perform each function involved in fat burning. These functions include:

- Increasing metabolism (improving calorie burn)
- Regulating blood sugar levels and minimizing insulin resistance
- Regulating hormone production and levels (ensuring cortisol and other fat-retaining hormones are kept in check)
- Improving the communication between the digestive system and the brain via neurotransmitters to ensure feelings of satiety are experienced appropriately

If you add turmeric to your daily diet, the essentials required for each of these processes are delivered to the proper organs via the bloodstream, promoting the successful functioning of each system. When each system is optimized, you'll find that your:

- Food is properly digested
- Bile production is balanced
- Energy levels are higher
- Feelings of fullness come easier
- Calorie-burn rates are higher

All of these benefits lead to increased fat burn, as verified in a *Journal of Nutritional Biochemistry* article in 2015! You can be sure your systems are optimized by incorporating turmeric into your day. With turmeric's blend of vital vitamins, miraculous minerals, and potent phytochemicals, the body's natural processes involved in fat burning are supported and optimized. Turmeric tastes great in teas, smoothies, snacks, and meals, so it's a very versatile and delicious ingredient that can maximize flavor *and* fuel fat burn. So, if you're hoping to lose fat without the pills, potions, and products that promise but don't deliver, opt instead for the natural doses of turmeric that can help you lose fat fast and healthfully!

18. TASTES GREAT IN A FAT-BURNING SMOOTHIE

This smoothie boasts thermogenic properties, thanks to the cayenne pepper, as well as all of the benefits that turmeric brings to the table.

TO MAKE THE FAT-BURNING SMOOTHIE, COMBINE IN A BLENDER:

1 cup water

½ cup lemon juice

1 mango, chopped

1 teaspoon powdered turmeric

1 teaspoon cayenne pepper

1 tablespoon pure maple syrup

Blend on high until all ingredients are thoroughly combined.

RECOMMENDATIONS FOR USE:

Sip once a day.

19. BOOSTS ENERGY LEVELS

If you find yourself fighting fatigue on a regular basis, turmeric may be able to help. In order to produce energy, the body breaks down nutrients like carbohydrates, proteins, and fats to deliver the specific components of each to corresponding cells that utilize the macronutrients for the production of adenosine triphosphate (ATP). ATP is a nucleotide triphosphate used within the cells for coenzymatic reactions that produce and provide energy.

Without going into the scientific background of energy production pathways, the important takeaway is that each pathway's efficiency is boosted with the addition of thermogenic foods like turmeric and other spices. Thermogenic foods (spicy foods, for example) raise the body's temperature above normal and also require additional energy expenditure in order to return the body's temperature to normal. This thermogenic process and additional energy output require the metabolism to work harder, the body to burn more calories, and all of the body's systems to work collectively in an effort to return the body's temperature and affected processes to normal.

Turmeric improves energy production in a number of ways:

- Its plentiful B vitamins help the brain's abilities to produce energy-sustaining biochemicals.
- Turmeric protects and improves immunity to ensure that the body doesn't succumb to illness and disease.
- Its ability to regulate blood sugar makes turmeric a powerful combatant against diabetes-related conditions, and helps keep energy levels stable.
- With the improved enzymatic activity and bile production stimulated by the curcumin in turmeric, the body can also experience an increased metabolism of the macronutrients, helping to improve the pathways of all energy production!

TO MAKE A TROPICAL TURMERIC ENERGY DRINK, COMBINE:

1 cup coconut milk
½ cup chopped pineapple
1 banana, peeled
1 teaspoon powdered turmeric
1 cup ice

In a blender, combine coconut milk, pineapple, banana, turmeric, and ½ cup ice. Blend on high until all ingredients are thoroughly combined. Add remaining ½ cup of ice gradually while blending until desired consistency is achieved.

20. REDUCES LDL CHOLESTEROL WHILE IMPROVING HDL CHOLESTEROL

Cholesterol has a bad reputation because most people think only of the bad form of cholesterol and the consequences of it that wreak havoc on health. The truth is that cholesterol is a necessary element of the diet that helps multiple systems by composing part of the outer lining of cells. Cholesterol only starts producing negative health conditions when the low-density lipoproteins in LDL cholesterol, commonly referred to as "bad cholesterol," build up in the blood and stick on the inner lining of arterial walls. This buildup then creates blockages that impede or completely inhibit blood flow altogether. Normal total cholesterol levels are below 200 mg/dL, and most people can maintain that level with proper diet, exercise, and lifestyle habits. Want to keep cholesterol levels in check naturally without the need for medication? Turmeric can help!

According to a 2008 study published in the *Archives of Physiology and Biochemistry*, vitamins, minerals, phytonutrients, and fiber in turmeric are able to ensure that the digestive system, cardiovascular system, and lymphatic system work synergistically to absorb necessary cholesterol while ridding the body of excess. Specifically, the curcumin within turmeric provides the body with an antioxidant that actually prevents LDL levels from rising by:

- Improving liver metabolism of cholesterol
- Scavenging cholesterol more efficiently from the blood
- Increasing fat metabolism rates to impede cholesterol buildup within cells

Who knew? A simple tablespoon of turmeric per day can help keep cholesterol at bay . . . naturally and deliciously!

21. CLEANSES THE LIVER

Your liver is tasked with the difficult job of cleansing your body's fluids of toxins, pollutants, and irritants. The liver therefore plays a major role in maintaining the body's immunity and its ability to fight infection and preserve overall health. If the liver itself is compromised with toxins derived from the diet, environment, or lifestyle choices, it functions poorly, and that can lead to catastrophic consequences that can adversely affect your body and mind. With a focus on healthy living, anyone can reverse damage done to the liver, improving its health and productivity.

With a fully functioning, healthy liver, the body and mind can thrive, free of oxidative properties and free radicals that can run rampant, killing or mutating cells throughout the body. (Oxidation is a process that produces harmful and potentially dangerous "free radicals" that can move throughout the body via the bloodstream and tissues, causing potentially harmful changes to cells.) Turmeric's cleansing phytochemicals act as powerful antioxidants and anti-inflammatory agents, protecting and cleansing the liver and the entire body!

TO MAKE A BEET AND TURMERIC SMOOTHIE, COMBINE:

1 red beet, peeled and greens removed

1 carrot

1 kale leaf

1" gingerroot, peeled

1 tablespoon powdered turmeric

1 tablespoon lemon juice

¼ teaspoon cayenne pepper

2 cups purified water

½ cup ice

In a blender, combine all ingredients except ice. Blend on high until all ingredients are thoroughly combined. Add ice gradually while blending until desired consistency is achieved.

RECOMMENDATIONS FOR USE:

Sip daily to protect and cleanse your liver.

22. INCREASES YOUR BODY'S ANTIOXIDANT LEVELS

Oxidation is a process that produces harmful and potentially dangerous "free radicals" that can move throughout the body via the bloodstream and tissues, causing potentially harmful changes to structures and cells. Antioxidants are potent molecules that inhibit the oxidation of other molecules and cells. Your body uses antioxidants to protect, preserve, and promote its health and well-being. Antioxidants come from numerous sources, with the most predominate being your diet. Vitamins A, C, D, and E are specific vitamins that do "double-duty" as antioxidants.

Turmeric is just one food that can add a surprising number of nutrients and antioxidants to the diet. Curcumin acts as a powerful antioxidant, combating free-radical damage, oxidative stress, and even the development of tumors and metastasizing cancer growth, according to a 2013 peer-reviewed scientific research study in *Redox Biology*. Adding delicious spice to any smoothie, snack, or dish, you can provide your body with a host of powerful antiaging, anticancer, antioxidative compounds that work to scavenge the brain and body of potential harm, replenish those areas with nutrition, and ensure their safety from future illness and disease.

TO MAKE A TASTY TURMERIC-BERRY TUMBLER, COMBINE:

1 cup blueberries

1 cup strawberries, tops removed

1 banana, peeled

½ cup spinach

1 tablespoon powdered turmeric

1 tablespoon organic honey

1 cup ice

In a blender, combine all ingredients except ice. Blend on high until all ingredients are thoroughly combined. Add ice gradually while blending until desired consistency is achieved.

RECOMMENDATIONS FOR USE:

Drink daily.

23. STIMULATES NUTRIENT ABSORPTION

Most of the body's nutrient absorption takes place in the digestive tract. Your body is able to reap the benefits of countless macronutrients (carbohydrates, proteins, and fats), vitamins, minerals, and phytochemicals from your daily dietary intake of foods and liquids. The extent to which the body is efficiently able to absorb these nutrients dictates how much of that nutrition is actually available for use. If your body is able to absorb only a fraction of those nutrients, you aren't reaping the whole-body benefits of all the good foods you eat. Turmeric helps improve your body's ability to absorb nutrients more efficiently in a number of ways, strengthening overall health naturally. Curcumin, the active compound in turmeric, boosts nutrient absorption by:

- Improving liver functioning as a result of eliminating toxins, reducing the number of free radicals, and lowering bad cholesterol levels in the bloodstream
- Improving digestion through reducing inflammation within the digestive system and hindering the growth of harmful bacteria that can impede nutrient absorption
- Increasing bile production, thereby improving enzymatic reactions that are essential in the breakdown, storage, and utilization of nutrients

Gain all of these benefits by adding just 1 tablespoon of tasty turmeric per day to your diet!

24. FIGHTS H. PYLORI

Helicobacter pylori (also known as H. pylori) is an extremely harmful bacterium found in the stomach that, surprisingly, is unknowingly carried by more than 50 percent of the population. Unlike the "good bacteria" that live in the digestive system to break down foods, H. pylori does the exact opposite: It can cause irritations, infections, and even cancer. Some people who have the bacteria never see any symptoms. But with an overgrowth of any one of the H. pylori strains, peptic ulcers and even stomach cancers can quickly develop, leaving the digestive system, immune system, and thus the entire body open to infections of all kinds.

Turmeric comes to the rescue, yet again, to help prevent this debilitating bacterium from hurting your health, while also providing preventative and restorative benefits for the future!

Curcumin goes into a protective and restorative mode, helping to kill off the existing strain(s) of H. pylori and prevent future overgrowths. Turmeric can also help heal the ulcers and precancerous or cancerous cells that developed from an H. pylori infection.

If you think you might have an H. pylori strain in your body, talk to your doctor and ask if eating a tablespoon of turmeric per day could help you!

25. SOOTHES SORE THROATS

Whether the underlying issue is a bacterial or viral infection, or a condition like heartburn or indigestion, sore throats can be uncomfortable and difficult to treat. Chemical-laden over-the-counter treatment options like sprays, cough drops, and lozenges may only manage symptoms temporarily, if at all, and they also deliver synthetic materials to an already compromised immune system. Instead, consider natural treatment methods that not only soothe symptoms but also work to fight the underlying causes. One of these unique natural treatments is, of course, turmeric.

Turmeric's antimicrobial, antibacterial, and antiviral compounds are able to provide the body with potent phytochemicals that directly attack the source of the sore throat . . . whether it be a mild infection or more serious illness. The best part? A study published in *Clinical Interventions in Aging* in 2014 showed that 1,500 mg of turmeric per day provides analgesic effects comparable to 800 mg of ibuprofen. The fact that turmeric also has anti-inflammatory properties, directly relieving the site of a sore throat, only amplifies the natural benefits that this unique spice can deliver to treat and soothe sore throats safely, effectively, naturally, and deliciously!

TO MAKE A THROAT-SOOTHING DRINK, COMBINE:

1 tablespoon grated turmeric
1 cup coconut milk
1 teaspoon honey
1 teaspoon cinnamon

Serve warm or at warm temperature.

RECOMMENDATIONS FOR USE:

Drink at least once daily while dealing with a sore throat.

26. ADDS KICK TO HOMEMADE CURRY POWDER

Homemade curry powder is usually milder than many of the store-bought versions. Old or stale curry powder can be dry-roasted in a pan to revive the flavors. If you'd like to add earthy tones to your favorite dishes, you can add a teaspoon or two of powdered turmeric to your ingredients as you wrap up the cooking process; not only will this ensure the antioxidants remain undamaged by heat exposure, the turmeric will maintain a minimal flavor that won't overpower the taste desired from the dish. Providing an astounding number of health benefits, this thermogenic addition will also help speed up metabolic functioning and improve immunity naturally.

TO MAKE HOMEMADE CURRY POWDER, FOLLOW THESE INSTRUCTIONS:

1 tablespoon black peppercorns
3 tablespoons coriander seeds
2 tablespoons cumin seeds
1 tablespoon cloves, whole
15 white Thai cardamom pods
2 tablespoons ginger powder
¼ cup turmeric powder
3 dried long Thai chilies or dried long New Mexico chilies

Toast each spice separately in a dry frying pan over low heat until fragrant. Cumin seeds will take about 1 minute, while the rest of the spices take about 2 minutes.

Combine all ingredients in a coffee grinder, working in batches if necessary. (Yields ½ cup.)

RECOMMENDATIONS FOR USE:

Store in a jar with a tight lid for up to 3 months. Use in any recipes calling for curry powder.

27. BOOSTS FLAVOR IN A SHRIMP PASTE RELISH

This dish is easy to make, and you can adjust it to your preferred taste. Adding a subtle spiciness to the relish, turmeric not only improves the inherently earthy flavor of the shrimp paste but also adds a delightful fragrance and color, making it appealing to all of the senses. The simple addition of turmeric maximizes nutrition content with valuable vitamins and minerals, while also providing astounding antioxidants that help promote and protect the body and all of its systems.

Alternatively, add all ingredients to a small food processor. Grind until blended. (Yields ½ cup.)

RECOMMENDATIONS FOR USE:

Serve with fish and fresh vegetables.

TO MAKE SHRIMP PASTE RELISH, FOLLOW THESE INSTRUCTIONS:

5 cloves garlic

1 teaspoon powdered turmeric

⅛ teaspoon salt

1 tablespoon shrimp paste, roasted

3–5 Thai chilies, red or green

2 teaspoons palm sugar

1 tablespoon lime juice

1 teaspoon fish sauce

Pound garlic, turmeric, salt, and shrimp paste with a mortar and pestle. Add chilies and pound until chilies are bruised and broken into smaller pieces. Season with palm sugar, lime juice, and fish sauce.

28. LIVENS UP MEAT IN A SWEET AND SOUR SAUCE

This sauce is thick, sweet, and sour, with a touch of spice. With a focus on whole, clean ingredients that add nutritional benefits and flavor, this recipe enhances the natural flavors of meat with a sweet and spicy kick. Plus, it includes only ingredients that promote health and well-being—without preservatives and additives that are commonly found in the store-bought varieties of sauces. The addition of turmeric helps to enhance the colors and flavors of your favorite dishes while benefiting the brain and body . . . deliciously.

TO MAKE A SWEET AND SOUR SAUCE, FOLLOW THESE INSTRUCTIONS:

1 tablespoon minced fresh long red chili (serrano, jalapeño, or finger pepper)
1 teaspoon minced garlic
1 teaspoon powdered turmeric
½ teaspoon salt
1 tablespoon sugar
½ cup organic, unfiltered apple cider vinegar

Combine all ingredients in a small saucepan. Bring to a boil over medium-high heat, then turn down to low heat and simmer until thickened, about 5–7 minutes. Remove from heat. (Yields ½ cup.)

RECOMMENDATIONS FOR USE:

Use atop any grilled meat, especially grilled chicken, steak, or seafood.

29. PERFECTLY SEASONS A BEEF SALAD WITH TURMERIC DRESSING

This is a classic Thai street food usually served with sticky rice. The dressing recipe is great for any type of grilled meat. Most Thai salads are spicy. The dressings almost always have a perfect balance of salty, sweet, sour, spicy, and bitter.

TO MAKE A BEEF SALAD WITH TURMERIC DRESSING, FOLLOW THESE INSTRUCTIONS:

Salad

1 pound rump roast

2 tablespoons soy sauce

3 cups mixed greens or shredded romaine lettuce

½ cup sliced pickling cucumber

½ cup cherry tomatoes

Handful of chopped cilantro

Dressing

4 fresh red or green Thai chilies, minced

4 cloves garlic, minced

3 tablespoons fish sauce

4 tablespoons lime juice

1 teaspoon honey

1 teaspoon powdered turmeric

1 teaspoon sugar

Marinate beef with soy sauce and let sit for 30 minutes.

Grill to desired doneness. Slice beef and put in a salad bowl. Throw in the rest of the salad ingredients.

To make the dressing, crush chilies and garlic with a mortar and pestle to a coarse paste. Add fish sauce, lime juice, honey, turmeric, and sugar to the chili and garlic paste. Alternatively, put all ingredients in a food processor or blender and blend until chilies and garlic are chopped into small pieces, about 10 seconds.

Add dressing to salad mixture and toss well. (Serves 4.)

RECOMMENDATIONS FOR USE:

Eat for lunch one day a week.

30. PROVIDES A QUICK LUNCH IN THAI SHRIMP CEVICHE

Thai Shrimp Ceviche is a famous restaurant dish. Turmeric not only adds a delightful golden hue to the meal, but provides antioxidant benefits to improve the immune system and safeguard cell health naturally. Make sure to buy fresh saltwater shrimp from a store you can trust. This dish is simply raw: As the shrimp sits in the lime juice, the protein is denatured. The shrimp appears cooked after being exposed to the high acidity.

TO MAKE THAI SHRIMP CEVICHE, FOLLOW THESE INSTRUCTIONS:

6 fresh red or green Thai chilies, minced

4 cloves garlic, minced

1 teaspoon powdered turmeric

3 tablespoons fish sauce

4 tablespoons lime juice

2 tablespoons chopped cilantro

1 pound medium-sized shrimp, peeled and deveined

Mix all ingredients, except shrimp, in a small bowl. Adjust ingredients to achieve the desired balance of salty and slightly sour.

Lay shrimp on a deep plate; pour dressing over shrimp. Place in the freezer for 20 minutes, then serve. (Serves 4.)

RECOMMENDATIONS FOR USE:

Eat for lunch one day a week.

31. ADDS FLAVOR AND COLOR TO A COOL SIDE DISH OF CUCUMBER SALAD

This easy dish is great as a side for several meals, especially dishes that contain dried spices like yellow curry or satay. Turmeric boosts the flavor of and adds a slightly earthy, spicy kick to this cool cucumber salad all while improving nutrient absorption. Including only clean ingredients, this salad provides immense nutrition—and turmeric enables the body to better absorb that nutrition for improved functioning of the brain and all of the body's systems.

TO MAKE CUCUMBER SALAD, FOLLOW THESE INSTRUCTIONS:

Dressing

⅓ cup white vinegar

⅓ cup sugar

½ cup water

1 teaspoon salt

Salad

3 pickling cucumbers

1 whole serrano pepper

1 thinly sliced shallot

1 teaspoon minced ginger

1 teaspoon minced turmeric

¼ cup chopped cilantro

In a medium saucepan, bring white vinegar, sugar, water, and salt to a boil to dissolve sugar. Turn off heat and let cool.

Quarter cucumber lengthwise and slice it thinly. In a mixing bowl, combine all ingredients and toss well with dressing. Let the salad rest for 20 minutes before serving. (Yields 4 cups.)

RECOMMENDATIONS FOR USE:

The dressing for this salad can be made way ahead of time. It will keep for several weeks in the refrigerator.

32. MARINATES CHICKEN SATAY

This appetizer or snack originated in Indonesia but has been largely influenced by Indian cooking styles. A perfect harmony of dry spices, fresh cilantro roots, and flavorful fish sauce, you'll find yourself turning to this mouthwatering dish again and again.

Peanut Sauce

2 tablespoons vegetable oil

⅓ cup coarsely ground peanuts

1 tablespoon sugar

1 tablespoon red curry paste

1 cup coconut milk

½ teaspoon salt

1 tablespoon lime juice

Chicken

8 ounces boneless, skinless chicken breast, cut into thin strips about 1" × 4"

¼ cup coconut milk

2 tablespoons chopped cilantro roots or stems

½ teaspoon curry powder

½ teaspoon turmeric powder

2 teaspoons sugar

1½ teaspoons fish sauce

2 tablespoons vegetable oil

Bamboo skewers

To make the peanut sauce, heat a saucepan over medium heat and add oil. Add peanuts, sugar, and curry paste when oil is hot, and fry at medium-low heat until fragrant, being careful not to burn the curry, about 15 seconds. Add coconut milk and salt.

Bring the ingredients in the saucepan to a boil. Boil for a few minutes or until the sauce thickens slightly. Adjust the seasoning with lime juice. The sauce should taste slightly sweet followed by a touch of tartness and saltiness. Cover to keep hot.

Marinate chicken pieces with coconut milk, cilantro roots or stems, curry powder, turmeric powder, sugar, fish sauce, and vegetable oil for 3 hours or overnight. Mix well with hand or spatula.

Soak bamboo skewers in water for 1 hour to prevent the skewers from burning.

Slide each slice of marinated chicken onto a bamboo skewer.

Grill skewered chicken until done and still moist, about 1½ minutes on each side. Serve hot with peanut sauce for dipping. (Serves 4.)

Serve this dish with a side of Cucumber Salad for a refreshing accompaniment.

33. ENHANCES A PASTE FOR CHICKEN IN PANDAN LEAVES

Pandan is a tropical plant used in Southeast Asian cooking. It is used like vanilla in desserts to add flavor and aroma. It is also used in many savory dishes and to make specialty drinks. In Thailand, this dish is a welcome treat when you go out to eat at restaurants.

TO MAKE CHICKEN IN PANDAN LEAVES, FOLLOW THESE INSTRUCTIONS:

3 skinless, boneless chicken thighs (or chicken breasts if preferred)
1 teaspoon minced cilantro roots or stems
⅛ teaspoon salt
2 garlic cloves, minced
1 teaspoon minced ginger
1 teaspoon minced turmeric
1 whole star anise
1 teaspoon ground white pepper, or 10 whole peppercorns
½ cup Thai sweet, thick soy sauce
5 tablespoons palm sugar
2 tablespoons light soy sauce
3 tablespoons Chinese cooking wine
2 tablespoons sesame oil
3 tablespoons water
12 pandan leaves
3 cups vegetable oil for deep-frying
1 tablespoon toasted white sesame seeds

Cut chicken into bite-sized pieces, about 3–4 pieces from one chicken thigh and about double that amount for chicken breasts.

Make a paste from cilantro roots or stems, salt, garlic, ginger, turmeric, star anise, and ground pepper or peppercorns using a mortar and pestle.

In a mixing bowl, mix sweet soy sauce, palm sugar, light soy sauce, Chinese cooking wine, and sesame oil. In a separate bowl, mix half of the sauce with all of the paste. Marinate chicken pieces with the paste-and-sauce mixture for at least 3 hours or, better yet, overnight in the refrigerator.

Make a dipping sauce by combining the other half of the sauce with about 3 tablespoons of water.

Wrap each chicken piece in a pandan leaf by placing chicken pieces toward the end of the leaf, leaving 2" of open space below the chicken. Grab the top of the leaf and start folding it around the chicken until about 5" are left, and then slide the remaining part of the leaf under one of the wrapped leaf sections to lock it in place.

Deep-fry in vegetable oil at 350°F and garnish with sesame seeds. (Yields 12 pieces.)

34. CHANGES UP A BORING STIR-FRY

This is a simple dish that is actually quite versatile. Keep in mind that you can change up the vegetables if you'd like, depending upon the availability during certain seasons, but be sure to add the vegetables that take longer to cook first. The staples of a stir-fry can be delicious . . . or quite bland. With the addition of a slightly warm and spicy ingredient like turmeric, the flavors of the meat, vegetables, and spices are enhanced, helping to naturally improve the flavor of stir-fries while adding a delightful color and bountiful health benefits!

TO MAKE A TURMERIC STIR-FRY, FOLLOW THESE INSTRUCTIONS:

2 tablespoons vegetable oil

2 garlic cloves, minced

8 large shrimp, peeled and deveined

½ cup sliced carrots

1 cup chopped asparagus, cut into 2" pieces

½ cup snow peas

2 tablespoons chicken stock or water

1–2 tablespoons light soy sauce

1 teaspoon turmeric, minced

Pinch of sugar

Pinch of ground pepper

Heat a wok over high heat until hot and add oil. Add garlic and fry over medium heat until fragrant, about 10 seconds. Add shrimp and stir-fry until shrimp just turn pink, about 1 minute.

Add carrots and stir-fry for 1 minute. Add asparagus and snow peas and sauté for another 2 minutes until vegetables are almost done. Add stock, soy sauce, turmeric, and sugar and fry for another minute. Serve sprinkled with pepper. (Serves 4.)

RECOMMENDATIONS FOR USE:

Visit your farmers' market and browse around to see what you can use for vegetables in this recipe. When substituting vegetables, think about textures and flavors that are similar to the ones you are substituting.

35. SPICES UP SUPER CITRUS SMOOTHIES

While few people might think of turmeric as the perfect smoothie addition, the delightful golden spice actually adds a subtle, slightly spicy kick to sweet smoothies. With this sensational blend of citrus fruits and coconut milk, turmeric not only intensifies the variety of flavors, but also boosts the health benefits! Adding to the citrus fruits' vitamin C, vitamin E, and bromelain are turmeric's potent phytochemicals and antioxidants. A delicious blend of energizing and immunity-improving nutrients and antioxidants comes pouring out of every last drop of this super citrus (and turmeric!) smoothie.

In a large blender, combine the pineapple, orange, grapefruit, turmeric, ice, and 1 cup of the coconut milk.

Blend on high until all ingredients are emulsified and thoroughly combined.

Add remaining ½ cup of coconut milk gradually while blending until desired consistency is achieved.

RECOMMENDATIONS FOR USE:

Start off your day with one of these smoothies for breakfast or a midmorning snack.

TO MAKE A SUPER CITRUS SMOOTHIE, FOLLOW THESE INSTRUCTIONS:

1 cup cored and chopped pineapple

1 orange, peeled and deseeded

½ pink or red grapefruit, peeled and deseeded

1 tablespoon turmeric

½ cup ice

1½ cups coconut milk

36. BOOSTS ANTIOXIDANT BENEFITS OF GREEN TEA

Green tea is well known for its natural provisions of potent antioxidants that help to safeguard the body's cells and systems from free-radical damage, illness, and disease. By infusing green tea with ginger and turmeric, the antioxidant benefits are improved immensely. Ginger provides its unique oil, *gingerol*, while turmeric adds its own phytochemical, *curcumin*, to every last drop of this delicious green tea blend, taking the health-protecting properties of green tea to new heights of natural health protection *and* deliciousness!

TO MAKE A GINGER- AND TURMERIC-INFUSED GREEN TEA, FOLLOW THESE INSTRUCTIONS:

1 gallon of water
2 (2") pieces of ginger, peeled and sliced
2 (2") pieces of turmeric, peeled and sliced
8 organic green tea bags

In a large pot over high heat, bring the gallon of water to a rolling boil.

Remove pot from heat and add ginger, turmeric, and green tea bags. Cover and allow to steep in a cool, dark place for 8–24 hours.

RECOMMENDATIONS FOR USE:

Drink at room temperature or over ice, and store in the refrigerator for up to 7 days.

37. ADDS COLOR AND FLAVOR TO WALDORF SALADS

Legend has it that the Waldorf Astoria of New York City first debuted the famous "Waldorf Salad" in 1893, and since then the delightful sweet salad has been improved upon in countless ways by countless chefs and cooks. In this delicious version, turmeric not only adds a beautiful golden hue and depth of flavor to the salad, but also increases the health benefits with curcumin's potent antioxidants. Delicious and nutritious, this Waldorf Salad is surely to be a staple in your recipe book!

TO MAKE A WALDORF SALAD, FOLLOW THESE INSTRUCTIONS:

¼ cup Greek yogurt

1 tablespoon lemon juice

½ tablepsoon powdered turmeric

1 cup chopped grilled or baked chicken

1 small red apple, cored and chopped

½ cup golden raisins

½ cup halved seedless red grapes

½ cup sliced celery

¼ cup chopped walnuts

2 heads chopped romaine lettuce

In a large salad bowl, combine Greek yogurt, lemon juice, and turmeric, and whisk until well blended.

Add chicken, apple, raisins, grapes, celery, and walnuts to yogurt, and toss to coat. Add chopped romaine, and toss until thoroughly coated.

RECOMMENDATIONS FOR USE:

Cover and chill for 1–2 hours before serving.

38. RELIEVES HEADACHES

Almost everyone gets a headache sometimes. From a dull ache to an excruciating pain, headaches run the gamut in terms of frequency, severity, and source. With accompanying symptoms that can include nausea, dizziness, sensitivity to light and sound, and even a disruption in thought patterns that can render the sufferer without focus, energy, or mental clarity, headaches can leave someone feeling helpless and victim to pain and discomfort for up to days at a time. Headaches are normally a result of a multitude of physical reactions in the body—such as dehydration, abnormal hormone levels, inflammation, and even disrupted nervous or cardiovascular system activity. Because turmeric can ward off these conditions, it's a perfect choice.

Turmeric's nutrients and phytochemicals act synergistically to support the body's natural processes. Turmeric acts specifically as a headache aid by moving through the digestive system, organs, and throughout the body to:

- Combat inflammation
- Restore hormonal balance
- Improve brain activity and nervous system communication
- Deliver natural analgesic compounds that help to fight pain naturally

All of these benefits combine to ensure that the body's natural processes return to normal. Turmeric therefore addresses both the causes of the headache (such as inflammation) and the symptoms that can accompany it (such as pain).

TO MAKE A HEADACHE-RELIEVING DRINK, COMBINE:

8 ounces water or coconut milk
1 teaspoon minced or powdered turmeric

RECOMMENDATIONS FOR USE:

Drink every few hours until symptoms subside.

39. MANAGES ARTHRITIS PAIN

Arthritis is pain and inflammation that occurs within the joints. Millions of people suffer from this excruciating condition, seeking relief in physical therapies, medicine, and lifestyle changes. While many things can be done to minimize the pain of arthritis, such as receiving cortisone shots, following daily prescription medicine regimens, and taking painkillers, the underlying cause of the inflammation is rarely affected. All of those treatments still leave the arthritis sufferer with "flare-ups"—aggravated further with synthetic pharmaceutical drug use that can wreak havoc on the body by interfering with normal functioning of the body's systems. Mood swings, interrupted sleep patterns, and heart complications are just a few of the commonly experienced side effects of pharmaceutical medications intended to treat arthritic conditions. By opting for a turmeric regimen, an arthritis sufferer can find relief from the condition effectively, safely, and naturally.

In a study on knee osteoarthritis published in *Clinical Interventions in Aging* in 2014, 1,500 mg of turmeric consumption daily was shown to have anti-inflammatory and analgesic properties comparable to 800 mg of ibuprofen. That's how turmeric is able to provide relief from arthritis pain while treating the underlying cause: inflammation. Helping to alleviate inflammation within the joints, turmeric's phytochemicals also work to cleanse the blood of impurities while promoting proper functioning of the liver to ensure that the toxins that can contribute to arthritis flare-ups are minimized throughout the body or are no longer present. All while delivering essential nutrients to improve the physical functions that help restore and replenish the health of joints throughout the body, turmeric might enable arthritis sufferers to enjoy a life without the condition and its limitations—naturally!

TO MAKE AN EASY ARTHRITIS PAIN RELIEVER, FOLLOW THESE INSTRUCTIONS:

1 cup water
1 green tea bag
1 teaspoon powdered turmeric
1 teaspoon powdered ginger
1 tablespoon organic honey

In a cup or small pot, bring water to a boil over high heat. Add green tea bag, turmeric, ginger, and honey, and steep for 10 minutes.

RECOMMENDATIONS FOR USE:

Drink 1–3 times per day for optimal results.

40. BATTLES RESPIRATORY INFECTIONS

Respiratory infections can be a result of a number of pathogens that are ever-present in our environments. Pollutants, allergens, bacteria, viruses, and microbes are constantly looming in the air, on surfaces, and even within the body—the contributing factors to the development of a respiratory infection are countless. With a properly functioning immune system, the body can easily fend off the development of most of these infections, but sometimes one gets through.

Because it contains a plethora of nutrients that provide the body with essential vitamins and minerals, turmeric supports the body's immune system, digestive system, cardiovascular system, and respiratory system by:

- Using its anti-inflammatory properties to open the airways and minimize breathing difficulties
- Improving blood flow and oxygen delivery to the lungs
- Clearing the body of toxins
- Maximizing immunity
- Acting as an antibacterial, antiviral, and antimicrobial agent

TO MAKE A LUNG-CLEARING DRINK, COMBINE:

1 teaspoon grated or powdered turmeric

1 teaspoon organic honey

8 ounces water or coconut milk

RECOMMENDATIONS FOR USE:

Drink 3–6 times per day to fight respiratory infections and restore the health of the systems of the body that will keep the respiratory system running as intended . . . without illness or disease!

41. LOWERS THE RISK OF HEART DISEASE

Heart disease is one of the deadliest conditions the population faces today, killing more people annually than any other disease. Heart disease (also known as cardiovascular disease) can strike individuals of any age, race, or gender . . . oftentimes without any warning. It can raise blood pressure, produce irregular heartbeats, contribute to the development of plaque and blockages in the arteries, and disrupt the normal functioning of the heart in a number of ways. Heart disease can also silently create health conditions of all kinds (such as stroke, heart failure, and heart attacks) or even death. With symptoms like chest pain, shortness of breath, pain in the neck and upper back, and numbness or tingling in the extremities, cardiovascular disease can easily be dismissed as isolated incidents of injury or fatigue, making the disease a silent killer. A focus on healthy living that includes a diet of clean, whole foods, combined with regular exercise and healthy lifestyle choices, can help anyone improve their chances of avoiding cardiovascular disease. Consuming turmeric can safeguard the body naturally, too!

With cleansing properties from the potent phytochemical curcumin, turmeric is able to prevent cardiovascular disease and promote heart health by:

- Scavenging the blood of impurities
- Improving cholesterol levels
- Regulating blood sugar levels
- Maintaining the proper functioning of the systems that contribute to the health of the cardiovascular system

TO MAKE A SIMPLE HEART-HEALTHY DRINK, COMBINE:

1 teaspoon grated or powdered turmeric
8 ounces water or coconut milk

RECOMMENDATIONS FOR USE:

Drink daily to keep cardiovascular issues at bay.

42. MINIMIZES THE THREAT OF COLON/ COLORECTAL CANCER

According to the American Cancer Society, an estimated 135,000 Americans are diagnosed with colon/rectal cancers every year, and about 50,000 will die from them. While the world's population has grown increasingly aware of cancers and the dangers these diseases pose to the entire body, colon cancer has not received nearly as much attention as others. Because colon cancer can be treated successfully if caught early enough, the World Health Organization and Centers for Disease Control and Prevention are trying to educate people on the identification, diagnosis, and prevention of colon cancer. Many people can avoid colon cancer successfully with a healthy diet, proper exercise, regular physician visits, colonoscopies, and awareness of symptoms such as rectal bleeding, chronic constipation, and discolored stools. With the implementation of turmeric in the daily routine, the chances of remaining cancer-free can be improved even further. How?

Curcumin, the starring phytochemical of turmeric, acts to prevent colon cancer in two astounding ways:

1. Its anti-inflammatory benefits minimize irritation and inflammation within the colon.
2. Its antioxidants combat cancerous changes in the body's cells. (Curcumin has been observed to fight free-radical damage and safeguard cells against the development of cancer and prevent possible metastases throughout the body.)

While promoting the health of the entire immune system and protecting against illness and disease that can leave the body vulnerable to cancerous changes, turmeric works diligently to prevent colon cancer successfully . . . and naturally! Add turmeric to your meals, or simply consume it in its fresh, powdered, or pressed form for better health and protection against colon cancer.

43. CAN HELP PREVENT ALZHEIMER'S DISEASE

A disease that affects an estimated 44 million people worldwide, Alzheimer's has a devastating effect on the human body. Alzheimer's halts working neurons, eats away at existing brain tissue, and wreaks havoc on the entire nervous system. Despite awareness and research, Alzheimer's is still considered an unpredictable and uncontrollable disease. We do know that the condition, which affects the masses, is exacerbated by the use of synthetic additives that are often included in food ingredients and storage containers, but we know very few preventative or curative measures at this point in time. However, recent scientific studies, such as a 2008 study published in the *Annals of Indian Academy of Neurology*, have shown how all-natural phytochemicals like curcumin could transform the treatment approach with fewer side effects and improved results!

The blood-brain barrier is an extremely selective permeable barrier that separates the circulating blood from brain fluid in the nervous system. This barrier blocks large molecules that can pose potential harm from interrupting the normal functions of the brain, nerves, etc. Unlike medicinal therapies that are unable to pass through the blood-brain barrier to deliver the caustic drugs directly to the brain sites affected by Alzheimer's, turmeric allows the potent phytochemical curcumin to be absorbed in the blood and delivered directly to the sites of the brain in need. Not only does curcumin fight inflammation and infection, this phytochemical combats protein deposits and nervous system inhibition by excavating these potentially hazardous protein deposits that contribute to the brain degradation associated with Alzheimer's disease. With a simple teaspoon of turmeric per day, grated fresh or in powdered form, mixed into meals, smoothies, or a simple elixir, you can help combat Alzheimer's disease naturally and deliciously.

TO MAKE A COCONUT-CURCUMIN TONIC, FOLLOW THESE INSTRUCTIONS:

1 cup coconut milk
1 teaspoon powdered ginger
1 teaspoon powdered turmeric
1 teaspoon honey

Heat coconut milk in a microwave-safe cup for 1–2 minutes, or until heated thoroughly.

Stir in powdered ginger, turmeric, and honey until powders and honey are dissolved and thoroughly combined.

44. FIGHTS MS SYMPTOMS

Multiple sclerosis is a terrifying disease that slowly degrades the myelin sheath of the neurons to the extent that the brain is no longer able to communicate with the muscles. Multiple sclerosis affects approximately 2.5 million people around the world, rendering the sufferers unable to communicate, move, or keep memory skills functional. With communication and mobility limited, multiple sclerosis patients are often unable to execute normal daily life skills. While the disease has been researched extensively over the past two decades, there is still no known cause, nor has a cure been discovered. But turmeric has shown to be helpful in relieving the symptoms.

Turmeric has been studied in numerous clinical trials (such as a 2009 study published in *The International Journal of Biochemistry & Cell Biology*) and has been shown to effectively minimize symptoms of fatigue, dizziness, blindness, and muscle tremors, as well as the breakdown in motor skills so often associated with the disease. With a simple dose of 50–100 mg of turmeric per day, patients observed showed a massive improvement in all symptoms—the progression of the disease was even halted in some cases. Multiple sclerosis sufferers can potentially find relief and regain the ability to enjoy life just by adding 1 teaspoon of turmeric to their diet!

45. DIMINISHES THE RISK OF PARKINSON'S DISEASE

With no known cause or cure, Parkinson's strikes millions around the world, rendering them unable to perform everyday tasks the average person takes for granted. This progressive disease takes its toll on the neurotransmitters responsible for muscle functioning, producing symptoms like tremors, muscle rigidity, loss of balance, and stooping in posture. Pharmaceutical medicines can unfortunately cause undesirable side effects, such as trembling, insomnia, loss of appetite, etc. The medical world has turned to turmeric for all-natural therapeutic alternatives . . . with success!

Turmeric has shown to be a successful deterrent in the progression of Parkinson's disease, thanks to curcumin's role as an antioxidant. Promoting anti-inflammatory, antioxidative benefits that help to support normal system functioning, turmeric has proven to be a safe, all-natural spice that helps to minimize the symptoms of Parkinson's. Unlike pharmaceuticals prescribed for treatment, turmeric's phytochemicals are able to cross the blood-brain barrier. That's how turmeric is able to potentially prevent the physical and biochemical interferences of oxidative stress, which may be responsible for the brain tissue and cell degradation that causes Parkinson's. So, add this delicious addition to your salads, smoothies, and favorite dishes to increase your resistance to this debilitating disease . . . naturally.

46. REDUCES THE RISK OF CANCER

Antioxidants are key to the topic of cancer resistance. With more than 100 types of cancer affecting an alarming percentage of the population every year, the American Cancer Society estimates one out of every four deaths can be attributed to this disease. Pharmaceutical companies promote chemotherapy products that can be effective but have debilitating side effects, so the natural remedies community has studied natural alternatives that can prevent the development of cancer and potentially even kill cancerous cells completely. Turmeric has been one of the natural remedies studied and has produced nearly miraculous results.

Combating chronic inflammation, a known contributing factor to the development of cancer, turmeric promotes the body's ability to fight the spread of cancerous cells. Its potent antioxidants support the body's natural immunity to oxidative changes— changes that can cause cancer to develop and progress. The Memorial Sloan Kettering Cancer Center has worked extensively to study the effects of turmeric on cancer development and has deemed it to be "one of the most effective cancer combatants," as reported in *Clinical Cancer Research*.

With the simple addition of 1 tablespoon of turmeric per day, you can naturally and effectively help to keep your body and mind clear of cancer.

47. IMPEDES CANCER METASTASIS

Cancer has the ability to metastasize, or spread to other sites, and move throughout the body with a rapid pace. As most of us know all too well, cancer can wreak havoc on the entire body, spreading to various cells of all systems and organs. According to the World Health Organization, 90 percent of cancer-related deaths are due to metastasis. With cancer being such an intensely progressive disease, the medical community has sought out a natural alternative to chemotherapies and medical intervention that often-times pose serious side effects, such as life-altering exposure to hazardous and harmful synthetic chemicals.

Turmeric has been used for centuries in Ayurvedic medicine, and we now know that it can help to stop cancerous cells from spreading throughout the body . . . effectively, naturally, and without side effects. Curcumin is able to help prevent the spread of cancer while also preventing the development of cancerous cells in the first place. With a simple addition of a single tablespoon of turmeric to your daily routine, you can try to prevent the metastasis of cancer naturally, without side effects, and while improving your overall health in countless ways.

48. HEALS BRUISES

Bruises are a part of life, but they can be unsightly and uncomfortable. Some people are more susceptible to bruising than others, and bruising can be difficult to prevent . . . and even more difficult to treat. People normally just assume that they have to simply wait for the bruising to subside. Surprise! There are natural methods to treat bruises, and turmeric is one of them!

With similar phytochemicals that mimic the effects of pineapple's potent bromelain, turmeric's unique curcumin acts to combat bruising effectively and naturally. Turmeric's potent antioxidants and its anti-inflammatory and anticoagulating compounds heal the wound and also work to clear out the dead blood cells and repair the original injury from the inside out. Without side effects of any kind, you can use turmeric orally or apply it topically.

TO MAKE A BRUISE-FADING COMPRESS, SOAK A FACECLOTH OR HAND TOWEL IN:

½ cup warmed water or aloe

Squeeze the cloth to release excess liquid, then coat with:

1 tablespoon powdered turmeric

49. ADDRESSES THE UNDERLYING CAUSES OF DEPRESSION

Millions of people suffer from depression every day. With varying degrees of this condition, it can be difficult to identify the best treatment for an individual patient. The pharmaceutical industry cleverly promotes medical treatments that generate an estimated $10 billion per year—in fact, medications intended to minimize depressive disorders are the most commonly sought-after prescriptions. Yet many of these medications fail to treat the underlying issues such as stress, anxiety, and biochemical imbalances in the brain and body, and these medications can produce startling side effects such as mood swings, insomnia, and even suicidal thoughts . . . making those initial issues far worse. Without aggravating the body with side effects and symptoms, turmeric comes to the rescue yet again.

In a 2014 randomized, double-blind, placebo-controlled study of fifty-six individuals with major depressive disorder by Adrian Lopresti, PhD, et al., of Murdoch University, Australia, in the peer-reviewed *Journal of Affective Disorders*, turmeric showed promise in alleviating depression. Turmeric supports the body's ability to manage depression by:

- Improving brain functioning
- Ensuring proper hormone development and distribution
- Maintaining communication within the brain and nervous system

If you suffer from depression, ask your doctor if turmeric could help you manage the disorder. A simple tablespoon consumed throughout the day in meals and snacks, or in powdered or pressed pill form, might be able to help you naturally without any side effects.

50. TREATS EYE INFECTIONS

Eye infections can strike anyone at any time, leaving an unsightly and uncomfortable condition that can be hard to treat. Even though medications and solutions promise to provide relief, many can actually worsen the infection. Riddled with synthetic additives, preservatives, and chemicals, prescription medications and over-the-counter treatments can cause undesirable side effects like pain, swelling, redness, and even temporary sight loss. Luckily, the natural medical community has determined turmeric to be a safe and effective alternative treatment.

Turmeric provides a wide array of compounds that combat the viruses, bacteria, and microbes that contribute to the development of eye infections. As an anti-inflammatory and analgesic phytochemical, curcumin also works to fight the pain, inflammation, and redness associated with the condition.

TO MAKE AN EFFECTIVE COMPRESS, COMBINE:

2 tablespoons powdered turmeric

1 tablespoon honey

1 tablespoon organic, unfiltered apple cider vinegar

1 cup warm water

RECOMMENDATIONS FOR USE:

Soak a facecloth in the mixture. Apply to the infected eye as often as needed to provide relief safely, naturally, and effectively.

51. IMPROVES YOUR QUALITY OF SLEEP

Insomnia is a chronic condition that strikes millions of people annually. A lack of sleep might not seem like a big deal, but it can cause irritability, mood swings, an inability to concentrate, mental fogginess, and dangerous levels of fatigue that make driving unsafe. You have probably heard of countless prescription medications intended to provide relief from sleeplessness—indeed, many insomnia sufferers opt for medical treatment. Unfortunately, these medications often don't work very well, and they can cause impairment of motor functions and cognitive abilities.

With turmeric, you might find an all-natural approach to achieving proper sleep patterns. Its chemical compounds support proper brain and nervous system functioning, improve blood flow, and maintain proper hormone balance. All of these benefits work to promote overall health while also improving the quality of your sleep. Natural relief for a better night's sleep!

TO MAKE A SLEEP-PROMOTING DRINK, COMBINE:

8 ounces warm chamomile tea or coconut milk

1 tablespoon honey

½ tablespoon powdered turmeric

RECOMMENDATIONS FOR USE:

Sip before bedtime.

52. KILLS MULTIPLE-MYELOMA CELLS

Multiple myeloma is an aggressive form of cancer that affects the plasma cells of bone marrow. This disease also adversely affects the white blood cells responsible for your body's healing powers by killing healthy white blood cells or causing oxidative damage that can wreak havoc on the entire body. With concerns of metastases to other parts of the body, multiple myeloma has been identified as an extremely progressive cancer that requires intense treatment. Chemotherapy, radiation, and multiple pharmaceutical therapies are often used to treat this cancer, but these remedies frequently produce harmful side effects that make treatment a horrible experience . . . and they damage healthy cells and tissue.

Frustrated with limited success in treating this condition, the alternative medical community sought to treat multiple myeloma effectively using natural ingredients. The Virginia Commonwealth University has found turmeric to be a safe and effective component of treatment for killing multiple-myeloma cancer cells.

53. SERVES AS A NATURAL PAINKILLER

Aches and pains of all kinds are a common occurrence in daily life, and therefore painkillers are packed into pocketbooks, medicine cabinets, and junk drawers. Promising to provide relief for almost every imaginable condition, these over-the-counter products often fail to live up to expectations and with continued, regular use can cause serious side effects, such as liver damage and adverse system functioning.

With the safety and efficacy of painkillers being questioned over the years, it's easy to see why people have sought out natural therapies. For centuries, Ayurvedic medicine has utilized natural ingredients to treat illnesses and conditions . . . including aches and pains. For stomachaches to swelling, headaches to back pain, acute to chronic issues, cultures around the world have turned to turmeric because of its potent pain-killing properties.

Turmeric's powerful phytochemicals reduce inflammation, stimulate the release of pain-killing hormones, and can be ingested or used topically. A study published in *Clinical Interventions in Aging* in 2014 showed that 1,500 mg of turmeric per day provides analgesic effects comparable to 800 mg of ibuprofen. No wonder it's been used for more than 4,000 years!

54. PROVIDES NATURAL ANTI-INFLAMMATORY AGENTS

Inflammation is a common cause of pain and discomfort, and can even contribute to the development of serious illnesses and disease. While many people opt to treat their inflammation with prescribed and over-the-counter anti-inflammatory drugs such as ibuprofen and NSAID pain relievers, these treatment options can fail to provide relief and pose serious health risks. For those with contraindicated conditions, or those taking prescriptions that can be interfered with by anti-inflammatory medications, an all-natural treatment option can provide safe, effective relief. Free of synthetics, and supported by scientific studies that have shown it to be free of side effects, turmeric is not only health-improving in a number of ways, it is as safe as it is effective.

Chemical compounds in turmeric, such as curcumin, combine with vitamins and minerals that support the body's natural processes of fighting inflammation. Potent and able to provide relief comparable to or exceeding that of synthetic alternatives (according to a 2014 *Clinical Interventions in Aging* article), turmeric can be used topically or orally to fight inflammation inside and out. Powdered turmeric, when dissolved in water and applied with a compress to the site of swelling, can provide immediate and long-lasting relief. Ingested orally in powdered or compressed pill form, turmeric can also prevent inflammation in the cells, tissues, and muscles . . . naturally and effectively. A topical solution can be applied as well to the site of muscle soreness, sprains, swelling, joint inflammation, and even general aches and pains! Best of all, these applications can be used as often as necessary to achieve relief naturally.

55. PRESERVES EYESIGHT

Degenerative eye diseases strike millions of people around the globe every year, rendering them helpless to a slow minimization of their ability to see. The sense of sight is one that can easily be taken for granted since most people are able to enjoy healthy eyesight or can address any deficiencies with corrective eyeglasses, contact lenses, or surgery.

Whether caused by genetics, injury, or simply old age, eye health can suffer in varied ways. Once considered a medical issue that was unpreventable, degeneration of the eyes is now known to be able to be improved with the addition of simple lifestyle changes: Not smoking, avoiding alcohol, engaging in regular exercise, and focusing on proper nutrition can all contribute to the maintenance and improvement of eye health. One of the nutritive additions that has shown to produce improvements is turmeric.

Effectively and naturally, turmeric can provide the eyes (and the supportive nerve systems involved with sight) with powerful phytonutrients that can protect against degeneration. Because it contains antioxidants; vitamins A, C, and E; anti-inflammatory compounds; and compounds that fight free-radical damage and oxidative stress that can degrade the eyes and optic nerves, turmeric is particularly beneficial to eye health. By consuming a simple teaspoon of turmeric daily in your diet, you can provide the eyes (and entire body!) with preventative and protective health measures naturally!

TO MAKE A SCRUMPTIOUS EYE-HEALTH SMOOTHIE, FOLLOW THESE INSTRUCTIONS:

2 carrots, tops removed
1 kale leaf
1 banana, peeled and frozen
1 teaspoon turmeric
2 cups purified water, divided

In a blender, combine carrots, kale, banana, turmeric, and 1 cup of water.

Blend on high, adding remaining cup of water gradually while blending until desired consistency is achieved.

RECOMMENDATIONS FOR USE:

Drink daily for optimum eye health.

56. MAINTAINS PROSTATE HEALTH

According to the American Cancer Society, approximately 200,000 American men will be diagnosed with prostate cancer every year, and a shocking 26,000 will die each year from the disease. An estimated one in seven men will receive the diagnosis at some point in their lives, making prostate cancer a significant concern for men around the world. Early detection plays a major role in receiving successful treatment for the disease, so prostate exams are highly recommended for men over forty.

Turmeric has shown to be an effective treatment for the symptoms and development of the disease. In a twelve-week, double-blind, placebo-controlled clinical trial cited in the *Journal of Cancer Science & Therapy*, a group of researchers determined that curcumin, the most potent of turmeric's phytochemicals, reduces symptoms associated with prostate cancer (such as urinary incontinence and infections) and that the spice's antioxidants produce a notable increase in cancer cell death. That's why turmeric is now widely recommended to minimize prostate cancer risk, especially within holistic health communities. The addition of just ½ teaspoon per day can help safeguard prostate health; doubling the dosage can help reduce the progression of prostate cancer.

57. RELIEVES ALLERGIES

Antihistamines are one of the most commonly prescribed and purchased medicines on the market. Allergy sufferers find themselves falling susceptible to uncomfortable symptoms, thanks to exposure to dust, dander, and environmental particles. Providing relief for the body's reaction to only a few specific allergens, however, these medications can't usually treat *all* symptoms, leaving the sufferer with conditions like difficulty breathing, irritated skin, and itchy or watery eyes that are associated with the allergic reactions from hard-to-treat allergens. The good news: your body's immune system is built to provide protection against allergic reactions, so it is possible to find relief effectively and naturally without medications.

According to a 2007 study in the *Journal of Clinical Immunology*, turmeric's curcumin and micronutrients act as antioxidants and anti-inflammatories to:

- Combat bacteria, viruses, and microbes for improved immune system functioning
- Combat the body's histamine responses—the very causes of allergic reactions

- Open the airways
- Improve the body's hormonal balance
- Block the inflammation that can result in itchy eyes, clogged sinuses, and mental "fogginess"

Turmeric can provide an all-natural allergy remedy without side effects.

TO MAKE AN ALLERGY-RELIEVING DRINK, COMBINE:

1 teaspoon powdered turmeric
1 tablespoon honey
1 teaspoon cinnamon
1 cup warm water, tea, or coconut milk

RECOMMENDATIONS FOR USE:

Drink once or twice daily while symptoms remain for a delicious allergy-fighting elixir that actually works!

58. BOOSTS IMMUNITY

You probably know that your immune system is responsible for protecting the body from the development of illness and disease. Few people realize, however, that a significant portion of the immune system is directly related to the digestive system. Ridding the body of waste while retrieving and absorbing essential nutrients from whole foods, the digestive system disperses the essential elements of the diet throughout the body. All of these benefits make the immune system function better, helping to keep the body free of bacteria, viruses, and microbes, as well as harmful oxidative damage from free radicals. With such importance being placed on nutrition for the body's optimal health, it's easy to see why the digestive system plays such an important role . . . making the quality of the diet consumed something that literally supports or degrades the body's immunity.

Knowing that nutrients such as vitamins, minerals, and phytochemicals support the body's immune system, researchers started delving into specific natural foods and spices that are especially good at maintaining, protecting, and boosting immunity. Turmeric has shown to be one of the best foods for this purpose. It provides the body with antioxidants; anti-inflammatory properties; and antiviral, antibacterial, and antimicrobial compounds. These benefits help to support the digestive system's ability to function at its best and also support the immune system's protective capabilities to keep illnesses and disease at bay. A simple addition of a small ½ teaspoon of turmeric to your daily diet can provide the body with these protective immunity-boosting benefits for greater health naturally.

59. CALMS CHEMOTHERAPY TREATMENT SYMPTOMS

Undergoing chemotherapy treatments can render cancer patients uncomfortable, weak, nauseated, exhausted, and riddled with pain. Turmeric, though, can potentially help cancer patients find relief in a number of ways. A 2002 study published in *Cancer Research* found that turmeric can indeed help, because:

- Its phytochemicals work to combat the growth of cancer cells, minimizing their development and killing them as well. Therefore, turmeric can help support cancer treatments by making them more effective.
- Curcumin's anti-inflammatory and analgesic compounds help to minimize the pain due to inflammation.
- Turmeric supports the digestive system with soothing and supportive nutrients to combat nausea, improve digestion, and boost the immune system support provided by the digestive system's components.
- Curcumin helps the brain and nervous system by encouraging an optimal balance of hormone production that can regulate mood,

minimize depression, and support the delivery of potent neurotransmissions throughout the body.

All of these benefits combine to possibly minimize the symptoms of chemotherapy while supporting the effects of treatment.

TO MAKE A CHEMO SYMPTOM–RELIEVING DRINK, COMBINE:

2 teaspoons powdered turmeric
8 ounces green tea or coconut milk

RECOMMENDATIONS FOR USE:

Drink daily to help ease symptoms.

60. MAY ASSIST WITH TUMOR REDUCTION

Tumors can develop in people of all ages, races, and both genders at any point throughout life. Most times, surgery and chemotherapy are the treatments used to give the patient the best chance at a positive outcome. Unfortunately, these treatments often take a long time and come with unpleasant and debilitating side effects. Tumors are often able to grow and metastasize throughout the body very quickly, so researchers, physicians, and patients alike are working hard to determine a treatment approach to tumors that can save the lives of millions around the world.

Turmeric has entered the research studies of countless institutes, showing promise in providing the medical community with just that: hope in finding a quick and effective approach to treating tumors. With an abundance of micronutrients and phytochemicals, turmeric has been studied in tumor therapy, showing success in halting development and in shrinking and curing tumors.

A 2009 research study reported by the Linus Pauling Institute in coordination with Oregon State University determined curcumin "may inhibit procarcinogen bioactivation and help prevent cancer by inhibiting the activity of multiple CYP enzymes in humans." Turmeric's phytochemicals have the capability to cross the blood-brain barrier and act as antioxidants, anti-inflammatories, and antitumoral agents (by inhibiting the growth of tumors and stopping the spread and growth of tumor cells). Turmeric has been shown time and again that it can kill cancerous cells, promote the re-growth and regeneration of cells, and restore and support the body's systems. Its ability to cleanse the blood of impurities and toxins that can further diminish the immune system helps the body fend off future illness and disease.

One simple teaspoon of turmeric per day can potentially help halt and hinder tumor development, safely, effectively, and naturally.

61. BALANCES HORMONE LEVELS

Hormones are involved in every imaginable process that takes place in the brain and body. Coursing through the body with ease, these hormones are necessary to support life functions of all kinds. Digestion, muscle contraction, nervous system functioning, sleep, and mood can all be attributed to a specific interaction of hormones, and that's why hormonal balance is so essential to quality of health and well-being. Researchers know that lifestyle factors and diet definitely play a major role in the maintenance of hormonal production and balance, but there are times when genetics and mutations throw off hormonal balance. While many drugs attempt to restore hormone balance, the scientific and medical communities have begun looking to natural remedies like turmeric for success without synthetics.

Turmeric is able to supply an ample amount of nutritive support to the body's hormonal production processes. Turmeric:

- Improves immunity by supplying phytonutrients that prevent illness, disease, and mutations that can hinder hormonal production
- Cleanses the blood of toxicity

- Crosses the blood-brain barrier for immediate on-site delivery of phytochemicals
- Regulates and supports the health of all organs involved in hormone production

One simple teaspoon per day of turmeric is an easy, safe approach to achieving hormonal balance.

TO MAKE A HORMONE-BALANCING SNACK, COMBINE:

1 teaspoon powdered turmeric
Avocado or banana slices
Chia or hemp seeds

RECOMMENDATIONS FOR USE:

Eat once a day for well-being benefits.

62. HEALS EARACHES

The ear is a direct passageway to the brain, allowing sounds of all sorts to carry important messages about our surroundings. The parts of the ear within the canal are very sensitive and require thoughtful care. Because many earaches and ear infections are due to a virus that won't respond to antibiotics, the holistic health community has urged sufferers to seek natural alternatives to prescription medications. Turmeric has succeeded as a treatment option yet again!

Able to combat bacteria, viruses, and microbes simultaneously with the same application, turmeric has shown to be an effective way to ease ear pain. In addition, turmeric's phytochemicals act as anti-inflammatory and analgesic agents to fight swelling, irritation, and pain. With absolutely no side effects, a simple turmeric elixir can be safely dropped into the ear canal with your doctor's okay. The solution cleanses the ear of dirt, diminishes pain, and returns the ear to a normal state effectively without the side effects possibly associated with synthetic alternatives. Even "natural" ear solutions can contain unwanted and unnecessary additives and preservatives, so using a homemade solution of turmeric can be the simplest and safest solution to solving ear issues while also providing immunity boosting and preventative nutrients . . . naturally.

TO MAKE AN EAR-SOOTHING SOLUTION, COMBINE:

¼ cup organic olive oil
1 teaspoon powdered turmeric

RECOMMENDATIONS FOR USE:

Apply 5–10 drops in the affected ear up to 5 times daily for 10-minute sessions until the pain subsides.

63. OFFERS MENSTRUAL PAIN RELIEF

Menstrual pain is a major issue for women around the world, and it can last for days or even weeks. Common symptoms include abdominal cramping (which can range from minor to severe); aches and pains that surge throughout the head, stomach, and genitals; sleep disturbances; and difficult-to-manage mood changes. Pharmaceutical companies offer prescription and over-the-counter remedies that promise to provide relief. Containing a plethora of questionable synthetic ingredients, these products are either designed for a wide range of symptoms (some of which you may not have) or fail to provide relief at all. Some products also come with side effects such as insomnia, grogginess, fatigue, weight gain, and further fluctuation in mood. It's no wonder that women worldwide have sought out a natural alternative . . . and found it, in turmeric.

Researchers have experimented with a number of natural alternatives and have found turmeric's specific blend of nutrients and compounds to be effective in treating menstrual pain. Turmeric:

- Provides anti-inflammatory and analgesic compounds that help to counteract the internal inflammation and pain
- Supports the digestive and cardiovascular systems, helping to improve blood flow and maintain proper digestion and immunity
- Helps regulate blood sugar levels and hormonal production, which control energy, sleep, and mood naturally

Safe and effective without side effects or unnecessary additives, a warm turmeric drink can provide relief to the cramping area as well as improve circulatory and hormonal benefits for optimal lasting relief. Plus, the tonic can be consumed as often as necessary to minimize menstrual pain naturally, day or night.

TO MAKE A CRAMP-RELIEVING DRINK, COMBINE:

1 teaspoon powdered turmeric
8 ounces warm green or chamomile tea
1 teaspoon honey

RECOMMENDATIONS FOR USE:

Drink whenever symptoms present themselves.

64. ALLEVIATES JAUNDICE

Jaundice is a condition most commonly seen in infants right after birth. The most common solution is placing the newborn under "bili lights," which help the condition subside. While jaundice is common among infants and children, once you move into adulthood, the exhibition of symptoms associated with jaundice can indicate serious underlying liver issues. Poor liver functioning can manifest in a multitude of physical symptoms that affect the color of eyes and skin (yellowing is the most common symptom of jaundice). Doctors can run a bilirubin test to confirm whether a patient has jaundice.

Turmeric is just one of the whole foods that can be used to combat jaundice naturally. As always, though, it is highly recommended that if you appear to have jaundice that you consult with a physician before starting any natural healing remedy. The phytochemicals of turmeric, especially curcumin, can have a natural improving effect on the liver, as can turmeric's antioxidants and essential nutrients like B vitamins and zinc.

A fully functioning liver ensures that excess toxicity of all kinds is properly flushed from the body. With a simple addition of a tablespoon of powdered turmeric to the daily diet, almost anyone can strive toward achieving the optimal healthy liver functioning that makes jaundice a condition of minimal concern.

65. MINIMIZES COLIC

Colic is a common condition experienced by a number of infants, toddlers, and children under the age of five. A growing number of "homeopathic" approaches have recently appeared in the form of syrups, salves, and tablets that promise to provide relief . . . yet rarely deliver the desired result. Because colic is usually a result of upset in the digestive system, cultures around the world have effectively treated the condition by focusing on improving the digestive system's functioning . . . with great success. One natural approach to healing the painful acid reflux thought to contribute to colic is the administering of turmeric. In many places around the world, caregivers add turmeric to baby bottles, meals, and children's drinks and smoothies to minimize colic naturally.

Turmeric's anti-inflammatory compounds counteract the digestive issues associated with acid reflux and restore a natural balance to the system. Promoting proper blood flow and delivering essential nutrients throughout the digestive system and the body, turmeric is able to calm colic quickly and efficiently without the concern of side effects.

Consult with your pediatrician prior to providing your child with any holistic or natural healing remedy to ensure that certain sensitivities or reactions do not occur.

BEFORE OFFERING THE FOLLOWING MIXTURE, TALK TO YOUR CHILD'S PEDIATRICIAN. TO MAKE A COLIC-CALMING MIXTURE, COMBINE:

1 teaspoon powdered turmeric
8 ounces water, breastmilk, formula, coconut milk, or almond milk

RECOMMENDATIONS FOR USE:

Drink once a day.

66. PREVENTS TOOTHACHES

Toothaches can result from infections and inflammation from any site—from the mouth to the sinuses to seemingly unrelated parts of the body such as the ears or upper neck! Over-the-counter products promise to provide relief, so consumers frequently turn to these chemical-laden products, which often simply mask the underlying issue that causes the toothache to begin with. The issue remains, though, that the underlying cause of the toothache, such as a bacterial, viral, or microbial infection, still festers.

Turmeric not only provides the body with a topical relief from the pain associated with the underlying infection but also administers potent phytochemicals that can kill the bacteria, viruses, or microbes responsible for the toothache. With curcumin as its star polyphenol, turmeric provides anti-inflammatory and analgesic benefits to calm the swelling and pain associated with toothaches, while additionally combating the health-compromising assailants of bacteria, viruses, etc., to prevent and protect against further infection.

TO MAKE A MOUTH RINSE, COMBINE:

¼ cup warm water

1 tablespoon powdered turmeric

RECOMMENDATIONS FOR USE:

Swish around the mouth several times a day to alleviate the pain of a toothache while also addressing the underlying cause.

PART 2

BEAUTY

Who knew that a simple spice like turmeric could transform your health *and* contribute to your beauty regimen? Adding turmeric to your beauty routine can help rejuvenate your skin, improve the look (and color!) of your hair, and fight signs of aging. With masks, moisturizers, and elixirs that utilize turmeric to add essential nutrition, powerful antioxidants, and potent phytochemicals, you can improve the look of your skin, hair, and nails naturally. This commonly used spice that has been a staple in culinary cuisine for centuries also has the ability to transform your body on the outside as well!

While many applications might seem very simple, the results of these turmeric concoctions are nothing short of astounding. Providing an abundance of vitamins and minerals, as well as unique phytochemicals and antioxidants, turmeric is a natural promoter of antiaging and rejuvenating solutions that can be applied to the skin, hair, nails, teeth, and more. If you can avoid the over-the-counter, synthetic products that are riddled with chemicals, produce undesirable side effects, and fall short in desirable results, why not opt for turmeric instead? Natural, holistic, and with centuries of proven success, this spice has helped to treat, improve, and cure countless conditions. This section will show you how turmeric can not only improve your health but recover your natural beauty, too!

67. SERVES AS AN INSTANT TANNING LOTION

Most people know that sun exposure can cause cancer and other skin conditions. Hundreds of products on the market limit the skin's absorption of harmful UV rays. While this healthier approach to maintaining the skin's health protects your skin in a number of ways, it can leave you lacking a sun-kissed glow that you might want. After all, a sunny glow indicates that you love outdoor activities and a healthy, vibrant lifestyle. For this very reason, many have chosen to keep their skin protected but also seek a healthy option to give their skin a touch of color.

The beauty market has recognized this want and provided a barrage of lotions, potions, and sprays that promise to deliver that desired tanned appearance, but many of these products contain harsh and harmful additives that can actually agitate the skin. The safest solution is the natural solution: using a combination of all-natural ingredients that can combine to nourish the skin while also adding a touch of color.

TO CREATE AN AT-HOME TANNING LOTION, COMBINE:

1 cup organic coconut oil in its liquid state
3 tablespoons powdered turmeric

RECOMMENDATIONS FOR USE:

Keep covered in a dark, cool place, and apply to the body as a nourishing cream twice a day.

68. PROMOTES NAIL HEALTH

The nails are a focus of beauty that generate billions of dollars of annual spending. Manicures, pedicures, polishes, and primping can add up quickly, and the beauty industry is well aware that consumers seek out and purchase products that will help them achieve long, healthy, strong, beautiful nails. While these products promise to promote nail growth and optimize nail health, few take into consideration that the synthetics, chemicals, and additives they're made of can actually undermine nail health. In addition, few consumers take into account that their diet can make a major impact on the health of their nails . . . after all, our nails' health and appearance starts from the inside, with nutrition promoting or degrading that health. Luckily, turmeric can be used both internally and externally to provide the nails with what they need to be strong, healthy, and beautiful naturally.

Adding 1 teaspoon of powdered turmeric to your daily diet can ensure that your nails receive iron, magnesium, potassium, and a variety of B vitamins—all of which work to build nail strength and health. Keeping the nails nourished and protected against bacteria and microbes that can pose health threats, while also delivering all-natural nutrients directly to the nails and nail beds, you can promote and preserve nail growth and health simply and easily.

TO MAKE A TOPICAL NAIL MASSAGE OIL, COMBINE:

1 tablespoon organic coconut oil

1 teaspoon powdered turmeric

1 teaspoon brown sugar

RECOMMENDATIONS FOR USE:

Massage the nails as often as necessary throughout the day. This oil will also exfoliate, thanks to the brown sugar.

69. TREATS ACNE

Acne is caused by a buildup of bacteria in the skin that gets trapped within pores and agitates the skin's surface. This buildup of bacteria produces unsightly bumps, pimples, boils, and cysts on and underneath the skin. When acne sufferers of all ages and genders seek treatment, it's often in the form of a prescription or over-the-counter medication that can pose additional risk to the skin. Because they often contain harsh chemicals and additives designed to cleanse the skin and clear pores, these treatments can further agitate, irritate, or even burn the skin's surface.

In order to treat acne *and* maintain skin health, researchers have found all-natural ingredients—such as coconut oil, lemon juice, and turmeric—to be just as effective as synthetic treatments but pose no risk to skin health. Without harm to the skin, these all-natural ingredients can be used on sensitive areas like the face and underarms, as well as those more resistant to irritation, like the chest and back. These ingredients come together to provide the skin with a nourishing provision of multiple nutrients while naturally combating bacteria and microbes that can wreak havoc on the skin's health.

TO MAKE A HOMEMADE ACNE TREATMENT, COMBINE:

1 cup organic coconut oil
1 tablespoon powdered turmeric
1 tablespoon lemon juice

RECOMMENDATIONS FOR USE:

Store in an airtight jar in a cool, dark place for up to 2 weeks. Use once every other day for normal skin, or daily for oily skin.

70. NOURISHES DRY SKIN

Predisposition to skin dryness, excessive washing, thermal conditions, and environmental factors can all produce itchy, dry, irritated skin. When the skin becomes excessively dry, it can be a constant nuisance. Because the condition is so prevalent, you can find hundreds of over-the-counter lotions, salves, and balms that can contain chemicals, synthetics, or additives to extend shelf life. These additions can actually worsen dry skin, causing it to itch, burn, or spread. Instead, think natural!

With an all-natural concoction of whole-food ingredients found right in your own home, you can have a constant supply of nourishing lotion that combats dry skin and provides relief for extended periods of time. Not only do these ingredients combat skin dryness upon application, but the nutrients and phytochemicals act together to restore optimal health to the skin to prevent future flare-ups.

TO MAKE A NOURISHING LOTION, COMBINE:

1 cup liquid avocado oil

1 tablespoon powdered turmeric

1 teaspoon honey

RECOMMENDATIONS FOR USE:

Store in an airtight jar in your refrigerator for up to 1–2 weeks. Apply the mixture as often as necessary, especially following bath time and before bed, to enjoy replenished and rejuvenated healthy skin free of dryness . . . naturally.

71. IMPROVES OILY SKIN

Oily skin strikes most people at some point in their lives. Skin can overcompensate with an excessive production of oils due to a number of factors:

- An overwhelming hormone imbalance
- Environmental conditions
- Excessive stress
- Unaccommodating lifestyle factors

Leaving a constant sheen on your face, oily skin can result in clogged pores or become a breeding ground for unwelcome bacteria. Products on the market to combat oily skin conditions often contain harsh acids and chemicals that can dry out the skin and leave the pH balance disturbed, leading to a cycle of overcompensating oil production and even more need for cleansers and oils designed to combat oily skin. With a change in diet and a homemade cleanser that can keep skin from becoming overly oily, anyone can combat oily skin naturally and safely without concern of chemicals and unwanted side effects.

Diet can improve your skin's ability to better regulate oil production, so you should focus on eating fresh fruits, vegetables, whole grains, and healthy fats, and avoiding foods high in sugar or unhealthy fats. Consuming 1 tablespoon of turmeric at some point during the day can help to improve the hormone production responsible for oil production—plus, it helps improve blood flow, metabolism, and digestion, all of which lead to healthier skin.

TO MAKE A HOMEMADE OIL-BALANCING CLEANSING MASK, COMBINE:

½ cup yogurt

3 tablespoons brown sugar

2 tablespoons lemon juice

1 tablespoon powdered turmeric

RECOMMENDATIONS FOR USE:

Store ingredients in an airtight jar with a tight-fitting lid, and keep in the refrigerator for up to 24–48 hours. Shake well to combine if ingredients separate between uses.

Apply mask to skin, allow to set for 10–15 minutes, and rinse thoroughly.

If the skin starts to tingle or develop an uncomfortable sensation, rinse immediately and reduce lemon juice by ½ to 1 tablespoon in the next batch.

72. REDUCES AGE SPOTS

Age spots are discolored patches on the skin that can result from excessive sun exposure, certain skin conditions, and environmental upset. These factors physically manifest as hyperpigmentation on the skin's surface. Scrubbing, harsh chemicals, and lotions designed to lighten the age spots can actually further agitate the spots and surrounding skin. While many products may promise to provide a solution for age spots, these products are often packed with synthetics and chemicals that can only worsen the condition and further compromise skin health. By opting for a natural approach, you can restore your skin's overall health from the inside out. Another option is to apply an all-natural topical turmeric remedy that cleanses and clarifies the skin while evening pigmentation and promoting blood flow to the areas in need.

Safe, effective, and all-natural, these two turmeric-based approaches will ensure that your skin is free of discoloration . . . naturally:

1. To keep your skin healthy from the inside out, include 1 tablespoon of powdered turmeric in your diet daily. A daily dose ensures that your body and skin are receiving adequate amounts of the necessary vitamins, minerals, and phytonutrients needed to promote skin health and alleviate underlying issues that may be contributing to the hyperpigmentation of the skin.

2. Try the following topical solution to treat exactly the areas you want to address.

TO MAKE A TOPICAL SOLUTION TO LIGHTEN AGE SPOTS, COMBINE:

2 tablespoons organic coconut oil
1 teaspoon powdered turmeric

RECOMMENDATIONS FOR USE:

Apply generous amounts of the oil to the age-spot areas as often as necessary throughout the day. You should begin to see results within 10–14 days. The mixture can be stored in an airtight container for up to 3–4 days.

73. LIGHTENS STRETCH MARKS

Stretch marks are silvery streaks that can appear on the skin's surface for a number of reasons: age, weight loss, weight gain, pregnancy, injury, etc. The products on the market designed to treat stretch marks are often targeted at women and have only minimal success or provide a multitude of possible side effects. In order to avoid the possibility of posing harm to the skin, a topical solution of coconut oil and turmeric can be used to lighten the appearance of stretch marks and provide a nutrient-rich base from which the skin can thrive and the skin's cells can regenerate and restore skin tone naturally.

Healthy medium-chain fatty acids (also known as MCFAs) provide the skin with protective qualities while helping to regenerate cells. In the following recipe, coconut oil combines with turmeric's and aloe vera's potent phytochemicals, which have been proven to promote blood flow and preserve skin-cell health while reducing the appearance of stretch marks.

TO MAKE A LOTION TO REDUCE UNSIGHTLY STRETCH MARKS, COMBINE:

½ cup organic coconut oil
2 tablespoons aloe vera
1 tablespoon powdered turmeric

RECOMMENDATIONS FOR USE:

Store in an airtight container in a cool, dark place. Apply as often as necessary in order to achieve safe and effective stretch-mark relief naturally within 6–8 weeks.

74. SOOTHES SUNBURNS

Sunburns can strike anywhere, from the sidelines of a ballgame to a day at the beach. Left unprotected, your skin can fall victim to the sun's strong rays, literally burning the top layers of the skin. This uncomfortable condition can actually turn to one of great danger, because cancer cells thrive when the skin has been exposed to oxidation. In an effort to soothe sunburns, many consumers purchase products that promise to relieve the discomfort and pain, but these only provide temporary topical relief. To protect your skin's overall health, the exterior layer of the skin is only the first of concerns that should be addressed. Following a burn, a topical solution of nutrient-rich ingredients is ideal to prevent cancers, promote skin-cell health, and safeguard the skin against possible infection.

Aloe has the ability to penetrate the skin's layers far better than any other topical ingredient, so a combination of aloe and turmeric can provide the skin with:

- Antioxidants that combat free-radical damage
- Anti-inflammatory compounds that fight irritation
- Analgesics that soothe pain naturally

Rich in phytochemicals that only improve the efficacy of the mixture, turmeric and aloe join forces to provide relief and protection from the health-degrading consequences of sunburns while improving the health of skin naturally.

TO MAKE A SUNBURN-SOOTHING BALM, COMBINE:

1 cup organic coconut oil
¼ cup aloe vera
1 tablespoon powdered turmeric
1 tablespoon honey

RECOMMENDATIONS FOR USE:

Store in an airtight jar in the fridge. Apply generously to burned skin as often as needed until the burn and pain subside.

75. EXFOLIATES SKIN

Many people suffer from lackluster skin, riddled with patches of dry or irritated areas. Even with a skin-care regimen that focuses on moisturizing, the healthy, supple appearance of skin can still remain elusive. The layers of dead skin cells that accumulate over the days, weeks, and years can become a layer that prevents the skin from being able to adequately absorb the moisturizing nutrients that can transform the skin's appearance. With a skin-care routine that focuses on removing dead skin cells, cleansing the skin, and *then* moisturizing, you can achieve the beautiful skin you desire.

By exfoliating the skin's surface, you give your skin a chance to absorb optimal nutrition that helps to promote skin health. In the scrub recipe that follows, turmeric combines with powerful natural ingredients—coconut oil, Epsom salts, and aromatic essential oil. These ingredients do a lot of jobs:

- Remove dead skin cells from the skin's surface
- Deliver detoxifying, antioxidant-rich, anti-inflammatory-rich, and phytochemical-packed nutrition
- Moisturize skin
- Offer a calming scent

TO MAKE AN EXFOLIATING SCRUB, COMBINE:

1 cup organic coconut oil

½ cup Epsom salts

4–6 drops lavender or eucalyptus essential oil

1 tablespoon powdered turmeric

RECOMMENDATIONS FOR USE:

Store in an airtight container for up to 2–4 weeks. In the shower or bath, gently rub the scrub over your skin in circular motions to remove dead skin cells. Rinse thoroughly to reveal soft, moisturized skin. Use daily to maximize results.

76. REPAIRS CRACKED HEELS

Cracked heels are an unsightly and painful condition that makes even the simplest tasks of walking or wearing shoes unbearable. While moisturizing can help rejuvenate the skin's surface, the rough, dry, and blistered or broken skin that is associated with this condition is hard to remedy with a simple moisturizer. Any open wounds become breeding grounds for bacteria, viruses, and microbes that can cause serious skin conditions far worse just than a cosmetic headache. By using a combination of gentle exfoliating ingredients that not only help to remove dead skin but also prevent infection and improve skin health, you can avoid using those store-bought abrasive skin removers, chemical-laden products, and ineffective moisturizers.

Along with brown sugar, which serves as a gentle exfoliant, coconut oil and turmeric combine to provide the heels with a sensitive-skin remover that gently softens roughness without irritation. Coconut oil and turmeric aid in the protection against irritation by delivering potent anti-inflammatory agents along with phytochemicals that act as antibacterial, antiviral, and antimicrobial agents to protect against illness and serious skin conditions. Skin rejuvenation and repair can begin with the first use, continuing to improve the skin's condition until the heels are fully repaired.

TO MAKE A CRACKED HEEL–REPAIR LOTION, COMBINE:

1 cup organic coconut oil
2 tablespoons aloe vera
¼ cup brown sugar
1 tablespoon powdered turmeric

RECOMMENDATIONS FOR USE:

Store in an airtight container for up to 2–4 weeks. Apply generously to heels, and use a washcloth to massage mixture on skin's surface. Repeat process twice daily as needed until skin is repaired and softened.

77. FIGHTS ATHLETE'S FOOT FUNGUS

One of the least-known aspects of all-natural ingredients like turmeric is that they possess potent phytochemicals that fight illness-causing agents of all sorts: Bacteria, viruses, fungi, and microbes stand no chance when antioxidant-rich ingredients like turmeric are introduced. That's right, turmeric is also able to fight fungi! Turmeric provides vitamins, minerals, and phytonutrients that combine to prevent, protect, and reverse uncomfortable and undesirable conditions like athlete's foot through both food and topical applications. By adding turmeric to your daily diet, you can introduce potent fungi-fighting phytochemicals that spread throughout the bloodstream and prevent infections from within. Not only does the curcumin in turmeric combat fungus-related conditions like athlete's foot from within, turmeric can be combined with other natural ingredients to create a topical solution as well.

A win-win for health both inside and out, turmeric provides relief while optimizing health safely, effectively, and naturally! As a delicious addition to your favorite meals, snacks, or smoothies, consume 2 tablespoons of turmeric daily—or simply take turmeric in powdered or pressed pill form—to ensure optimal health without the fear of undesirable side effects. You can also apply turmeric right to the feet to provide site-specific relief. Treating the pain as well as the underlying fungal cause of athlete's foot, the following application is an easy way to solve all athlete's foot issues naturally!

TO MAKE A TOPICAL ATHLETE'S FOOT TREATMENT, COMBINE:

1 tablespoon powdered turmeric

¼ cup aloe vera

¼ cup Epsom salts

¼ cup organic coconut oil

RECOMMENDATIONS FOR USE:

Apply generous amounts to the affected area of the feet. Allow the treatment to set for 15–30 minutes before rinsing. Repeat as often as necessary until the infection subsides.

78. REJUVENATES SKIN IN A PERSONALIZED FACE MASK

DIY face masks can be a holistic approach to healing and helping skin reach optimal health. Without the fear of the chemicals, additives, and synthetic preservatives used in over-the-counter masks, a make-it-yourself, at-home application is an inexpensive and simple approach to supplying your face with effective ingredients that provide astounding nutrients for amazing results. The best part? DIY masks have rich sources of vitamins, minerals, phytonutrients, and phytochemicals—and you can concoct them in your own kitchen using fresh ingredients that require nothing more than a glass jar with a tight-fitting lid and refrigeration. This turmeric-based mask offers many benefits, as it:

■ Fights bacteria that can cause acne
■ Regulates oil production from hormonal imbalance
■ Helps avoid excessive dryness from inadequate blood flow and moisture
■ Relieves redness from irritation and inflammation

Following are four variations that start with a base mixture of coconut oil and powdered turmeric so you can create the perfect face mask for your individual skin type quickly and easily.

TO MAKE A PERSONALIZED SKIN MASK BASE, COMBINE:

2 tablespoons organic coconut oil
1 teaspoon powdered turmeric

To that, add ingredients based on your individual skin type:

- **Oily skin:** Add 2 teaspoons organic, unfiltered apple cider vinegar—it helps dry up excess skin oil without drying out skin.

- **Dry skin:** Add 2 teaspoons organic honey and 1 teaspoon almond milk—these ingredients help restore moisture and improve skin's ability to retain moisture naturally.

- **Inflammation:** Add 2 tablespoons espresso powder, 2 tablespoons natural cocoa, and 1 tablespoon honey (dry skin) or lemon juice (oily skin)—espresso's and cocoa's naturally occurring phytochemicals help relieve inflammation.

- **Discoloration:** Add ½ cup fresh pumpkin pulp—the antioxidants contained in the pumpkin pulp help to restore proper pigmentation production and balance in the skin, and help to reduce blotchiness and discoloration.

Apply the mask to your face. Let set for 10–15 minutes, then gently wash off and blot dry with a towel.

Store the remaining mask mixture in the refrigerator, and discard after 5–7 days.

79. MOISTURIZES SKIN AT NIGHT

Nighttime moisturizers make up a big part of the lotions you see on store shelves. Seeping into the skin without the disruption of sweat, makeup, or environmental pollutants that can interrupt moisturizers during the day, nighttime moisturizers can provide extra relief from skin conditions, aging, and irritation without interference. With promises that vary from providing simple nourishment to skin toning to skin tightening, the products available can be a confusing array of options that often require purchasing and applying multiple products. Unfortunately, these frequently contain chemicals, synthetic additives, and a multitude of possible skin agitators, so over-the-counter moisturizers can make for more harm than good. Why not consider an all-natural alternative that focuses on including only whole, natural ingredients? An easy, at-home creation of moisturizing ingredients is the perfect facial or body moisturizer that can remain on the skin's surface throughout the night, providing only relief and benefits without the risk of any adverse side effects.

Turmeric contains many components that can work overtime at night:

- Antioxidants that combat signs of aging, cellular degradation, and various skin conditions
- Anti-inflammatories that fight redness and irritation
- An abundance of vitamins and minerals that help the skin remain looking young, supple, and vibrant

The following at-home nighttime moisturizer can be used every night on any area of the skin you desire.

TO MAKE A NIGHTTIME MOISTURIZER, COMBINE:

½ cup organic coconut oil

¼ cup aloe vera

1 tablespoon powdered turmeric

1 teaspoon liquid vitamin E

5–10 drops lavender essential oil (depending upon how strong you'd like the fragrance)

RECOMMENDATIONS FOR USE:

Store in an airtight container for up to 2–4 weeks. Apply generously to the face, neck, and chest before bedtime. Rinse in the morning. Use nightly for best results.

80. RELIEVES ECZEMA

Eczema is a common skin issue that can affect individuals from infancy through old age. With redness, itchiness, irritation, and even broken skin characterizing this condition, there's no wonder why sufferers would seek relief. Because eczema flare-ups can continue for weeks or months, many people turn to prescription or over-the-counter creams that promise to resolve the issue, but few are effective and even fewer can provide protection against the worsening of the condition or the infections that can result from broken skin and open wounds. Some prescriptions are steroids, which are very powerful but can wreak havoc on the skin and actually further agitate existing irritation. Clearly, a soothing, natural option might be a better choice for a lot of people.

Turmeric, coconut oil, and aloe vera team up in this lotion to supply potent anti-inflammatory phytochemicals that provide relief from inflammation and also allow for a natural analgesic effect that calms itching and burning. The coconut oil and aloe vera act as transporters that effectively penetrate the skin's layers, allowing the antioxidants and the antibacterial, antiviral, and antimicrobial benefits of the turmeric to resolve the underlying cause of the eczema while safeguarding the skin from future conditions that could arise from the irritation of broken skin.

TO MAKE AN ECZEMA SALVE, COMBINE:

½ cup organic coconut oil
2 tablespoons aloe vera
1 tablespoon powdered turmeric

RECOMMENDATIONS FOR USE:

Store in an airtight container in a cool, dark place. This mixture will keep for 2–4 weeks. Apply directly to the site of the eczema 2 times a day, or as often as necessary for pain and itch relief.

81. PREVENTS SKIN INFECTIONS

Skin infections are one of the most common types of infections simply because the skin is exposed to bacteria, viruses, and microbes of all kinds throughout the entire day. The constant barrage of toxins that the body is exposed to in any environment is absorbed through the skin, making it susceptible to illness, disease, and infection. Because antibiotic-resistant strains of germs have become more prevalent, an open wound of any kind can be a gateway to serious illness and disease. For this reason alone, many people have become more concerned and want to safeguard their health naturally. While store-bought solutions, such as handy antibacterial dispensers that tend to be overused, have become a common product for treating skin wounds and combating microbes that can spread easily, these products can actually make the body's natural defenses inferior. They minimize the body's exposure to naturally occurring microbes in the environment and lessen the immune system's natural workload that actually keeps it strong. This inadvertently allows for infections to take hold more easily, more powerfully, and without resistance.

Turmeric's antioxidant-rich curcumin can provide a number of preventative benefits while also promoting immunity and supporting skin health. Turmeric can:

- Prevent bacteria, viruses, microbes, and fungi from infiltrating a wound
- Ensure that the skin-cell regeneration process is safeguarded against the infiltration of illness and disease-causing oxidative reactions
- Moisturize skin naturally and safely

TO MAKE A PROTECTIVE LOTION, COMBINE:

½ cup organic coconut oil

2 tablespoons aloe vera

1 tablespoon powdered turmeric

RECOMMENDATIONS FOR USE:

Store in an airtight container in the refrigerator for up to 2–4 weeks. Use as often as necessary on any surface of the skin for relief and protection.

82. PROMOTES WOUND HEALING

Antioxidants have been shown to be powerful protectants against the oxidative processes that can wreak havoc on cells, transforming healthy cells into cancerous ones. Providing the ultimate protection against serious illness and disease, these antioxidants also promote general cell health and safeguard against degenerative processes that inhibit natural cellular functioning. Antioxidants like curcumin have exhibited an extraordinary ability to not only protect against infection and inflammation but also specifically support the body's ability to heal wounds—naturally repairing and restoring health to areas that have been adversely affected by burns, cuts, and sores.

A topical turmeric application adds enormous benefits to safeguard a wound from infections of all kinds. It provides:

■ Essential nutrients to help regenerate skin cells
■ Antioxidants to protect against cell degradation
■ Vitamins and minerals to support blood flow, oxygen delivery, and white blood cell production
■ Compounds to provide pain relief and infection protection while also promoting the regeneration of the skin

The coconut oil, aloe vera, and honey in the following cream support the delivery of these nutrients to the subcutaneous layers of the skin.

TO MAKE A HEALING SALVE, COMBINE:

½ cup organic coconut oil

2 tablespoons aloe vera

1 tablespoon honey

1 tablespoon powdered turmeric

RECOMMENDATIONS FOR USE:

Store in an airtight container in the refrigerator for up to 2–4 weeks. Apply to a wound on any surface of the skin (even an open wound) as often as necessary. Wrap with gauze to ensure the applied mixture stays in place and minimal exposure to environmental toxins is permitted.

83. RESTORES HANDS AFTER EXCESSIVE WASHING

Health professionals always recommend hand washing as a deterrent against contracting illness and infection. And with making regular trips to public restrooms, touching doorknobs, and being exposed to environmental toxins of all sorts, the average person *should* wash his or her hands regularly throughout the day. Yet most soaps, antibacterial solutions, and harsh alcohol-based hand applications cause dryness and irritation. If you want to wash your hands regularly but not live with the resulting irritation, try an all-natural solution that can be kept in a simple store-bought squirt bottle. You'll keep your hands free of microbes while also reaping moisturizing benefits.

Coconut oil has long been used as an intense moisturizer and when combined with aloe vera is able to penetrate the skin's layers more effectively. Turmeric's anti-inflammatory compounds and essential nutrients supply the skin with supportive vitamins, minerals, and polyphenols that not only provide skin cells with protection against oxidative stress but also promote their health and stability throughout the process of maintenance

and regeneration. The combination of all three ingredients—coconut oil, aloe vera, and turmeric—defends your hands against bacteria, viruses, microbes, and toxins in the environment, with the added benefits of sustained, deep-layer moisturizing that protects and promotes skin health.

TO MAKE A RESTORATIVE LOTION, COMBINE:

½ cup organic coconut oil

2 tablespoons aloe vera

1 tablespoon powdered turmeric

4–6 drops essential oil, such as lavender, eucalyptus, or lemon

RECOMMENDATIONS FOR USE:

Store in an 8-ounce squirt bottle. Apply to hands at any time throughout the day as often as needed.

84. SERVES AS A NATURAL ANTIBACTERIAL MOISTURIZER

The use of hand sanitizers has increased exponentially in the last decade, with consumers hoping to prevent infections by applying an alcohol-based sanitizer to their hands as often as possible. These over-the-counter, alcohol-based solutions pose their own set of problems, though: They kill naturally occurring, protective bacteria on the skin that is geared toward safeguarding against infection and illness. Repetitive use of these antibacterial hand sanitizers can actually diminish your natural immune defenses against illness and disease, allowing for infections and illness to occur more often.

Instead, look to turmeric. With the addition of turmeric to the daily diet and to a regular topical solution that can be applied to the hands and skin, anyone can naturally safeguard their immunity against the offenses of the microbes that constantly challenge the immune system. By adding just 1 tablespoon of turmeric to your daily diet, you'll help all of your body's systems work synergistically to combat the offenses of the daily toxins your body faces.

TO MAKE A TOPICAL ANTIBACTERIAL LOTION, COMBINE:

½ cup organic coconut oil
2 tablespoons aloe vera
1 tablespoon powdered turmeric
5–10 drops lavender, eucalyptus, or lemon essential oil

RECOMMENDATIONS FOR USE:

Store in an airtight jar. Use as often as necessary throughout the day.

85. MINIMIZES APPEARANCE OF SCARS

Scars are a natural result of healing, but they can be unsightly and bothersome to some people. The beauty industry has tried to emphasize how "ugly" scars can be—a campaign that is especially effective on many women. The solutions on the shelves are often laden with chemicals, synthetics, and additives; these products not only fail to deliver the expected results but can also have side effects that lead to irritation, inflammation, redness, or infection at the site of application. As an alternative to these scar-diminishing creams that come with such risks, many have sought out holistic healing therapies with only the most natural of ingredients . . . one of which is turmeric.

TO MAKE A SCAR-REDUCING CREAM, COMBINE:

½ cup organic coconut oil

2 tablespoons aloe vera

1 tablespoon powdered turmeric

RECOMMENDATIONS FOR USE:

Store in an airtight container for up to 2–4 weeks. Apply generously to the site of scarring as often as possible throughout the day (especially at bedtime when applications are less easily interrupted).

Applied areas can be wrapped with gauze to prevent staining and oily residues on clothing.

86. REDUCES BODY ACNE

Acne can appear as easily on your body as it can on your face. Bacteria flourish on the skin's surface at all times, and some skin types are more likely to have clogged pores and develop acne. Body acne can be just as embarrassing as facial acne. But skip the chemicals in store-bought options and try this natural solution.

Turmeric provides a protective and preventative front against the accumulation of harmful bacteria responsible for acne. With the use of turmeric in an all-natural, homemade mixture of whole-food ingredients, the delivery of optimal nutritive vitamins, minerals, and phytonutrients required by the skin can be naturally achieved, allowing the skin to achieve a healthy pH balance and providing the nutrients it needs to restore and repair acne-related issues.

RECOMMENDATIONS FOR USE:

Store ingredients in an airtight container, ensuring all ingredients are thoroughly combined. Apply generously at least twice per day for 10–15 minutes to skin sites prone to body acne, and then rinse thoroughly.

TO MAKE AN ACNE-CLEARING CREAM, COMBINE:

1 cup organic coconut oil
½ cup organic, unfiltered apple cider vinegar
2 tablespoons lemon juice
2 tablespoons aloe vera
1 tablespoon powdered turmeric

87. HEALS BURNS

It might seem impossible to find an all-in-one treatment for burns since burns vary in origin and degree of intensity. Over-the-counter topical treatments promise to deliver relief, but most just address the symptoms, not offering real skin repair.

In this salve, natural ingredients (coconut oil, aloe, honey, and turmeric):

- Provide phytochemicals, such as curcumin, that act as an antioxidants and anti-inflammatory, analgesic, and antimicrobial agents
- Support skin-cell regeneration
- Protect against infection and illness during recovery

TO MAKE A BURN-HEALING SALVE, COMBINE:

½ cup organic coconut oil

2 tablespoons aloe vera

1 tablespoon honey

1 tablespoon powdered turmeric

RECOMMENDATIONS FOR USE:

Store all ingredients in an airtight container. Apply to burn site, wrap with gauze, and repeat as often as necessary to restore health and support healing naturally. This salve can be stored in the refrigerator or in a cool, dark place for up to 4 weeks.

88. EXFOLIATES THE FACE

The skin on your face should be treated with the most delicate of care. This is exactly why facial exfoliation is such a hot topic among skin-care gurus. Some companies claim that chemicals, synthetic additives, and harsh abrasives are necessary to effectively remove dead skin cells; others are proponents of more natural processes that can be applied to achieve the same results. With the vast number of products on the market, natural and otherwise, claiming to provide the face with exfoliating benefits, it can be difficult to decide what is best for your skin. When it comes to facial exfoliants, though, it's always best to be careful.

In order to avoid adverse reactions to store-bought options, opt for an all-natural-ingredient, at-home combination. Try this simple recipe for a gentle exfoliating base, along with moisturizing benefits and plenty of nutrient-rich support that can help to maintain skin health while removing dead skin cells effectively and naturally.

TO MAKE A FACIAL EXFOLIANT, COMBINE:

½ cup jojoba oil
¼ cup brown sugar
2 tablespoons honey
1 tablespoon powdered turmeric

RECOMMENDATIONS FOR USE:

Store all ingredients in an airtight jar with a tight-fitting lid, and keep in a cool, dark place for up to 4 weeks.

Apply liberal amounts of the exfoliant to the face, and gently smooth the mixture across the top of the skin in small circular motions. Rinse thoroughly with warm water. Repeat once daily.

89. DIMINISHES WRINKLES

Wrinkle cream sales dominate the beauty industry, with billions of dollars being spent by consumers on wrinkle-prevention products every year. In an effort to purchase restorative potions, creams, and salves that can rejuvenate the skin and prevent the appearance of wrinkles, consumers fall victim to the creative marketing strategies of well-known skin-care companies but too often to no avail. With the focus on only results, the prevalence of chemical-laden wrinkle correctors and fillers have become commonplace, and consumers often don't realize that these widely accepted synthetics can negatively impact overall health.

The skin is the barrier between exterior environmental toxins and the bloodstream, so you have to be very careful about what you put on your skin. A study published in 2016 in *Advances in Skin & Wound Care* showed that phytochemicals help skin achieve the wrinkle-fighting results of potent synthetic chemicals. Natural phytochemicals, like curcumin and others found in turmeric, have been deemed to have the same skin reformative capabilities as non-natural alternatives.

TO MAKE AN ANTI-WRINKLE CREAM, COMBINE:

½ cup organic coconut oil
2 tablespoons aloe vera
1 tablespoon powdered turmeric

RECOMMENDATIONS FOR USE:

Apply twice a day. Keep in an airtight container with a tight-fitting lid for up to 2–4 weeks in a cool, dark place. You should see results in 4–8 weeks.

90. TREATS DANDRUFF

Any dry skin condition can be uncomfortable, but the dryness of the scalp that leads to dandruff can be embarrassing as well. While the condition is common, few people realize that the underlying issue may simply be the overuse of hair-care products that contribute to the dryness of the scalp and eventually lead to the production of dandruff flakes. A number of dandruff-resolving shampoos are available over the counter, but many contain harsh chemicals that can either exacerbate the underlying issue or agitate the scalp and leave hair looking dull, oily, or dry. Instead of these chemical-laden options, try the all-natural alternative of a turmeric shampoo, providing relief from dandruff while promoting the health of the scalp naturally.

Bountiful provisions of vitamins, minerals, and potent phytochemicals from turmeric allow this natural ingredient to improve scalp health while simultaneously restoring a natural balance to the skin for effective treatment of the underlying issue. Excessive dryness of the scalp is combated naturally with the moisturizing and restorative benefits of coconut oil and aloe vera.

TO MAKE A NATURAL DANDRUFF-REDUCING SHAMPOO, COMBINE:

1 cup organic coconut oil
½ cup aloe vera
2 tablespoons powdered turmeric

RECOMMENDATIONS FOR USE:

Soak the scalp with the mixture. Wrap head with plastic wrap or a hair covering, let set for 10–15 minutes, and then rinse thoroughly. Or, apply the solution in the shower and rinse out. There's no need to shampoo with regular products afterward.

Store in a room-temperature, dark place that allows the ingredients to stay in liquid form.

Use as often as necessary to promote scalp health, heal dryness, and prevent further development of dandruff.

91: PREVENTS HAIR LOSS

Hair loss can almost always be attributed to a nutritional deficiency. Whether the deficiency is due to a poor diet, lifestyle choices, or hereditary conditions, the failure of the body to absorb and utilize essential nutrients can adversely affect multiple physical processes, including the production and retention of hair. The hair follicles can be compromised, leading to a minimal production of new hair growth and inability to retain existing hair. Over-the-counter products that promise to prevent hair loss often include harsh chemicals and synthetic additives that can agitate the skin and inhibit the healthy, natural retention of hair. Surprisingly, using turmeric is one of the natural approaches to preventing hair loss.

Because it contains a number of nutrients that help the skin achieve an optimal level of health, turmeric can be used in both internal and external applications to ensure the scalp remains healthy and hair continues to grow. Aloe vera delivers essential nutrients, while leaving the hair free of residue or oily buildup. Fighting free-radical damage that can leave the scalp riddled with health issues, turmeric's polyphenols help to counteract the health issues and conditions that can cause hair loss.

TO MAKE A HAIR-RETAINING SOLUTION, COMBINE:

2 tablespoons turmeric

¼ cup organic, unfiltered apple cider vinegar

1 cup aloe vera

10 drops lavender or tea tree essential oil (optional)

RECOMMENDATIONS FOR USE:

Store all ingredients in a jar with a tight-fitting lid, and shake vigorously to ensure ingredients are thoroughly combined before using again.

Massage solution into the scalp and allow to set on the scalp for 15–30 minutes. Rinse thoroughly. Shampoo and condition as usual. Repeat daily for best results.

92. STIMULATES HAIR GROWTH

There's no question that the quality of nutrients (or lack thereof) in the diet can play a major role in the speed and health of new hair growth. If your body receives an abundance of essential nutrients like vitamins and minerals, as well as proteins, fats, and carbohydrates, the hair can respond by growing at a vigorous rate with strands that are healthy, vibrant, and strong. Split ends and breakage can occur with unhealthy strands lacking in key building blocks, like protein and biotin especially, so it is absolutely essential to include a variety of nutrient-rich foods in the diet to ensure the body and hair receive proper nutrition for the optimization of hair growth. The same process applies to the stimulation of new hair growth.

Turmeric is able to support the stimulation of new hair growth by providing nutrients and phytochemicals. Consuming 1 teaspoon of powdered turmeric daily can help improve the body's distribution of nutrients to the scalp and for the processes related to hair production. With the restored balance of hormones, blood supply, and metabolism due to better distribution of nutrients, the scalp and hair can benefit immensely, leading to the stimulation of new, healthier hair growth.

You can also make a topical solution to apply directly to your hair. Ridding the strands of buildup, stimulating circulation to the scalp, and providing nutrients directly to the scalp and hair, the topical solution provides even more support for healthy, natural, and safe stimulation of hair growth that actually works!

TO MAKE A CONDITIONER TO ENCOURAGE HAIR GROWTH, COMBINE:

1 tablespoon powdered turmeric
1 tablespoon organic, unfiltered apple cider vinegar
¼ cup aloe vera

RECOMMENDATIONS FOR USE:

Apply to the hair, massage into the scalp, and allow to set for 15 minutes before rinsing. Use once per day.

93. WHITENS TEETH

So many people want whiter teeth. Promising to improve the appearance of teeth, products available over the counter guarantee to whiten teeth by a shade or more. While these marketing ploys sound appealing, the chemicals and additives used to remove stains and whiten the teeth can be a major area of concern. Increased sensitivity, softening of enamel, and damage to the internal makeup of the teeth can all result from use of whitening products. These possible side effects can lead to a decline of the health and appearance of teeth in the future, so many consumers have sought more natural approaches to whitening that not only improve the appearance of their teeth but provide added health benefits as well.

"Pulling" is a mouth-rinsing process that has been used by cultures around the world for centuries. Swishing coconut oil can naturally remove bacteria, viruses, and microbes from your gums and teeth. Not only does this process help to rid the mouth of illness and disease-causing invaders, it can remove stains from the teeth as well. Adding turmeric to your daily coconut oil pulling ritual can:

- Provide antibacterial, antiviral, and antimicrobial phytochemicals
- Stimulate circulation
- Improve the calcification of the teeth
- Safeguard enamel strength for stain-fighting protection that lasts

That's right—improved health and whiter teeth from a simple mouth rinse of all-natural ingredients that can be found in your cabinet every day!

TO MAKE A TEETH-WHITENING PULL RINSE, COMBINE:

1 tablespoon organic coconut oil
¼ teaspoon powdered turmeric

RECOMMENDATIONS FOR USE:

Swish in your mouth for 10–20 minutes, 1–3 times per day.

94. NATURALLY BRIGHTENS HAIR

Thanks to environmental toxins, excessive use of hairstyling products, heat damage, and poor dietary nutrition, hair can take on a dull, lackluster appearance. Riddled with breakage; split ends; frizz; and deficiencies in essential proteins, fats, and amino acids, unhealthy hair can be an indication of internal unhealthiness that makes it nearly impossible to have hair that looks the way you want. While products on the market promise to help calm frizz, repair breakage, and restore a more moisturized, healthy appearance, the damage done to hair can be difficult to overcome permanently. But by adding turmeric to your daily diet as well as to a simple topical solution, you can start naturally repairing damage and restoring health to your hair today!

Turmeric provides a number of essential nutrients, all of which can directly affect the healthy growth of hair. It:

- Supplies B vitamins, proteins, fats, and amino acids that help build and maintain the strength of hair
- Improves blood flow to the scalp, helping to stimulate healthy hair growth

A simple tablespoon of turmeric added to the daily diet can help ensure that your nutrient needs for healthy hair are met every day. If you apply turmeric directly to your hair, you get the added benefit of delivering protective phytochemicals that help safeguard strands against toxins and even heat-and-styling degradation, improving the appearance of your hair for years to come!

TO MAKE A TOPICAL HAIR-BRIGHTENING SOLUTION, COMBINE:

¼ cup aloe vera

3 tablespoons fresh lemon juice

1 tablespoon organic, unfiltered apple cider vinegar

1 tablespoon powdered turmeric

RECOMMENDATIONS FOR USE:

Apply to the hair and allow to set for 15 minutes before rinsing.

95. TREATS SCALP CONDITIONS

Scalp conditions can arise from a number of health issues and can be difficult to treat. Bacteria, viruses, microbes, and fungi can all breed on the scalp, leading to conditions that can be unsightly and uncomfortable. In addition, products applied to the scalp can cause burning or itchiness and can transfer chemicals, additives, and synthetics to the bloodstream beneath the skin's layers far more easily than through the thicker layers of skin on other areas of the body. For this reason alone, you should take extra precautions when choosing a scalp-condition cure. Many treatments suggest leaving the product on the scalp for an extended period of time—all the more reason to be sure you use natural products. With a few simple, all-natural ingredients you have in your refrigerator and cupboard, you can make your own scalp treatment without the safety concerns that can result from the use of synthetic products.

Dryness, redness, irritation, and broken skin are all symptoms of common scalp conditions, and all can be treated with turmeric. The following scalp treatment offers these benefits:

- Anti-inflammatory, antibacterial, antiviral, antifungal, and antimicrobial phytochemicals
- Analgesic effects to calm itchiness and pain
- Moisturizing effects

TO MAKE A SCALP TREATMENT, COMBINE:

¼ cup organic coconut oil

¼ cup aloe vera

1 tablespoon turmeric

10 drops tea tree oil

RECOMMENDATIONS FOR USE:

Apply to the scalp for 15 minutes before rinsing, allowing the protective phytochemicals to penetrate the skin and provide relief. There's no need to shampoo with regular products afterward.

This rinse can be used as often as necessary until the condition has subsided, and can be used regularly for preventative use 1–3 times per week.

96. MOISTURIZES LIPS

Dry, cracked lips can be unsightly, uncomfortable, and a breeding ground for health-deterring bacteria, microbes, and viruses. You can find countless lip balms at the drugstore, but they contain synthetics, chemicals, and additives that sometimes do more harm than good. It can also be difficult to find one that's not flavored or overly scented.

Skip the chemical-laden lip balms on the market, and whip up an all-natural, at-home, nutrient-rich alternative in the comfort of your own kitchen. With natural anti-inflammatory and analgesic compounds, the following lip balm recipe can provide pain relief and reduce redness and inflammation naturally. It contains:

- Medium-chain fatty acids (MCFAs) from coconut oil that promote healthy system functioning
- Skin-penetrating polyphenols from aloe vera
- Phytochemicals from both turmeric and ginger that protect and promote health

What's not to love? This simple combination of natural ingredients acts to benefit your health while beautifying your lips.

TO MAKE A LIP BALM, FOLLOW THESE INSTRUCTIONS:

1 cup organic coconut oil

¼ cup aloe vera

1 tablespoon powdered turmeric

1 tablespoon powdered ginger

Mix well, then refrigerate for 24 hours until solid.

RECOMMENDATIONS FOR USE:

Transfer 2 tablespoons of the balm to a small container with a tight-fitting lid, and apply generously throughout the day and before bedtime.

This solution can be stored in the refrigerator for up to 3–4 months, while smaller amounts can be stored in a small container, to be carried in the car or purse, for 1–2 weeks.

97. COMPLEMENTS AN AROMATHERAPY PRACTICE

Turmeric has been used in culinary dishes, religious rituals, and cosmetics for centuries. This warm "golden spice" of the ages infuses experiences with a calming sensation and warm aroma that evokes feelings of peace and serenity. It might be surprising to learn that turmeric can also be used to stimulate the senses for increased energy and focus. Curcumin, the potent phytochemical in turmeric, works in a number of ways. It:

■ Benefits the circulatory system's blood flow
■ Targets the brain's hormonal production of dopamine and serotonin
■ Promotes nervous system functioning
■ Maximizes metabolic processes

These benefits can either provide calming stress relief or promote energy, depending on how and when you use turmeric. Helping to promote overall health, this spice can be used as an effective all-natural aromatherapy aid that not only helps to calm or energize but also penetrates the skin with essential nutrients that safely and effectively optimize health and well-being.

TO MAKE A PRESSURE-POINT OIL, COMBINE:

½ cup organic coconut oil

1 tablespoon aloe vera

1 tablespoon powdered turmeric

RECOMMENDATIONS FOR USE:

Apply to pressure points on the inside of the wrists, at the temples, and even behind the knees and on the bottoms of the feet to provide calming relief at bedtime, during meditation, or before a busy day of stress or to promote energy and focus before energy-requiring activities.

98. CLEANS AND PROTECTS TEETH

Consumers are bombarded with a dizzying number of toothpastes that promise to deliver a variety of benefits: protection against gum disease to reduction in sensitivity to whitening effects. Unfortunately, these well-marketed pastes often contain harsh chemicals and additives that can cause oral concerns, aggravate existing conditions, or deteriorate gum health and the composition of teeth. There's an all-natural alternative, though, that can be used as often as desired without the possibility of side effects: turmeric! With the simple addition of a sprinkle of turmeric on your toothbrush and toothpaste, you can easily add health-improving nutrients to your daily oral-hygiene routine. Turmeric's protective benefits naturally combat bacteria, viruses, fungi, and microbes, and may help protect against common health issues that can originate in the mouth. Gum disease can lead to other destructive illnesses and to disease-causing pathogens that can be distributed throughout the bloodstream and digestive system, but turmeric can also help prevent gum disease.

By using turmeric as a toothpaste, you can deliver the "golden spice's" benefits to your life by allowing them to be absorbed through the bloodstream and digestive system, making the absorption, metabolism, and processing of the nutrients even more effective. Turmeric toothpaste helps to:

- Whiten teeth
- Ensure enamel strength
- Prevent sensitivity and oral conditions of all varieties

Turmeric might just be the most effective aesthetic-improving addition to your daily beauty routine that also optimizes overall health. Just sprinkle some on your toothbrush, then brush and rinse normally.

99. MAKES A CALMING OR ENERGETIC BATH

Soaking in a warm tub of fragrant, moisturizing water and bath salts or bubbles can help promote feelings of calm and tranquility or rejuvenating and energizing stimulation. Depending upon your goal, you can transform your bath time to help you achieve feelings and sensual stimulation of all kinds. Instead of a plain bath or one doused in chemical-laden bubbles, consider an at-home solution of all-natural ingredients, so you can enjoy a safe, effective, sensual soak in the bath with moisturizing and health benefits!

With the addition of turmeric to your bath, you can soak up essential nutrients that promote skin health and optimize overall wellness. The following recipe contains powerful ingredients that bring many benefits to your bath:

- Turmeric's unique aroma stimulates the senses
- Coconut oil transforms your bath into a rejuvenating spa-like experience in the comfort of your own home
- Aloe adds moisturizing benefits and allows the turmeric to be better absorbed through the skin
- Coconut oil's MCFAs, polyphenols, phytochemicals, and essential nutrients effectively penetrate the skin's deepest layers

Able to combat the underlying causes of skin conditions that can begin with bacteria, viruses, microbes, and fungi, these ingredients help your bath time not only become a sensual experience that can calm, revitalize, and moisturize but also provide preventative benefits to help ensure skin health and safeguard internal health as well. So, utilize turmeric, coconut oil, and aloe vera for beautiful, supple, moisturized skin that lasts for days and is only a bath time away!

TO MAKE A BATH SOAK, COMBINE:

1 cup organic coconut oil

¼ cup aloe vera

2 tablespoons powdered turmeric

10–15 drops lavender or tea tree essential oil

RECOMMENDATIONS FOR USE:

Place a ¼–½-cup portion of the mixture on the bottom of the bathtub, and then start the hot water, allowing the coconut oil to melt and the aloe and turmeric to be evenly distributed throughout the bathwater.

100. CONDITIONS DYED HAIR

Hair dye can be one of the most toxic chemicals you can use on your body. With the chemicals, colorings, additives, and synthetics used to ensure hair dye achieves a desired effect and remains permanent through daily washings and other hair-care routines, hair dyes can wreak havoc on health. Applied to the hair and scalp, the chemicals contained in hair dyes can seep directly into the skin and bloodstream, allowing toxins to enter the body. These toxins, putting undue pressure on the blood, organs, and systems, can inhibit natural physical processes and contribute to the development of cellular degradation, illness, and disease. Luckily, an all-natural hair-health aid is available to help hair and overall health: turmeric.

Dyed hair strands can lack moisture and more readily absorb toxins from the environment and hair products, only exacerbating the issues posed to hair health and appearance. Turmeric's protective antioxidants, vitamins, minerals, and phytochemicals act as potent protective nutrients so that dyed hair can retain health and boast beautiful, moisturized locks of shine, volume, and bounce that most consumers can only hope to achieve. With essential nutrients that promote hair and scalp health, cleansing agents that remove residue naturally, and moisturizing phytochemicals that prevent dryness and protect against toxic infiltration of the hair's strands, turmeric, coconut oil, and aloe vera help to maintain a beautiful head of hair . . . naturally!

TO MAKE A CONDITIONER FOR DYED HAIR, FOLLOW THESE INSTRUCTIONS:

½ cup organic coconut oil

2 tablespoons organic, unfiltered apple cider vinegar

¼ cup aloe vera

Add all ingredients to a microwave-safe glass or ceramic jar. Microwave contents for 1 minute, or until thoroughly heated.

Shake or stir vigorously to ensure contents are well combined.

RECOMMENDATIONS FOR USE:

Apply solution to hair, coating strands thoroughly. Wrap with a shower cap or plastic wrap, and allow to set for 15–30 minutes. Rinse thoroughly and shampoo and condition as normally.

Repeat daily to ensure best results.

BIBLIOGRAPHY

Aggarwal BB, Harikumar KB. "Potential Therapeutic Effects of Curcumin, the Anti-inflammatory Agent, Against Neurodegenerative, Cardiovascular, Pulmonary, Metabolic, Autoimmune and Neoplastic Diseases." *The International Journal of Biochemistry & Cell Biology*. 2009;41(1):40–59.

Dhillon N, Aggarwal BB, Newman RA, et al. Phase II trial of curcumin in patients with advanced pancreatic cancer. *Clin Cancer Res*. Jul 15 2008;14(14):4491–4499.

He ZY, Shi CB, Wen H, et al. Upregulation of p53 expression in patients with colorectal cancer by administration of curcumin. *Cancer Invest*. Mar 2011;29(3):208–213.

Heck AM, DeWitt BA, Lukes AL. Potential interactions between alternative therapies and warfarin. *Am J Health Syst Pharm*. 2000;57:1221–1227.

Jagetia GC, Aggarwal BB. "Spicing up" of the immune system by curcumin. *J Clin Immunol*. 2007;27:19–35.

Kuptniratsaikul, V., Dajpratham, P., Taechaarpornkul, W., Buntragulpoontawee, M., Lukkanapichonchut, P., Chootip, C., Laongpech, S. (2014). "Efficacy and safety of Curcuma domestica extracts compared with ibuprofen in patients with knee osteoarthritis: a multicenter study." *Clinical Interventions in Aging*, 9, 451–458.

Lone, Jameel, Choi, JH, Kim, SW, Yun, JW. "Curcumin induces brown fat–like phenotype in 3T3-L1 and primary white adipocytes." *The Journal of Nutritional Biochemistry*, 21 September 2015.

Lopresti, Adrian, PhD, et al. *Journal of Affective Disorders*. 167(2014)368–375.

Mishra, Shrikant and Kalpana Palanivelu. "The effect of curcumin (turmeric) on Alzheimer's disease: An overview"; *Ann Indian Acad Neurol*. 2008 Jan–Mar; 11(1): 13–19.

Pari L, Tewas D, Eckel J. "Role of curcumin in health and disease." *Arch Physiol Biochem*. 2008;114:127–49.

Somlak Chuengsamarn, Suthee Rattanamongkolgul, Rataya Luechapudiporn, Chada Phisalaphong, Siwanon Jirawatnotai. "Curcumin extract for prevention of type 2 diabetes." *Diabetes Care*. 2012 Nov ;35(11):2121–7.

Thangapazham RL, Sharad S, Maheshwari RK. "Phytochemicals in Wound Healing." *Adv Wound Care* (New Rochelle). 2016 May 1; 5(5):230–241.

Trujillo, et al. "Renoprotective effects of the antioxidant curcumin: Recent findings," *Redox Biology*, 2013.

INDEX

ABOUT THE AUTHOR

Britt Brandon is a Certified Personal Trainer and Certified Fitness Nutrition Specialist (certified by the International Sports Science Association, ISSA) and Health Coach (certified by the American Council on Exercise, ACE) who has enjoyed writing books that focus on clean eating, fitness, and unique health-promoting ingredients such as apple cider vinegar, coconut oil, and aloe vera for Adams Media. In her time with Adams, she has published eleven books, including *The Everything® Green Smoothies Book*, *The Everything® Eating Clean Cookbook*, *What Color Is Your Smoothie?*, *The Everything® Eating Clean Cookbook for Vegetarians*, *The Everything® Healthy Green Drinks Book*, *The Everything® Guide to Pregnancy Nutrition & Health*, *Apple Cider Vinegar for Health*, *Coconut Oil for Health*, and *Ginger for Health*. As a competitive athlete, trainer, mom of three small children, and fitness and nutrition blogger on her own website (*www.ultimatefitmom.com*), she is well versed in the holistic approaches to keeping one's self in top performing condition . . . and actually uses turmeric daily in food and drinks, as well as in many home remedies.